MW01484274

How to Buy a Dental Practice

Brian Hanks, MBA, CFP®

ISBN-10:1544112114
ISBN-13: 9781544112114

CONTENTS

ABOUT THE AUTHOR

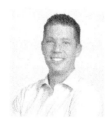 Brian Hanks, MBA, CFP® is an accountant and financial advisor for dentists. Brian has served the dental community at two dental accounting firms where he focused on newer dentists in transition. He has extensive experience working with dental transitions concentrating mainly on working with buyers of dental practices.

Brian is passionate about helping dentists develop great, lucrative, and rewarding careers. He frequently speaks on topics related to dental transitions, leadership, accounting and investments. He resides in the Mountain West and works with dentists across the entire United States.

ACKNOWLEDGMENTS

Thank <u>you</u> for reading this book. Buying and then reading another's words is an amazing gift. I appreciate the trust extended.

I'd also like to thank my dear wife Natalie, who has persevered with me across the country and throughout my career. Her encouragement was vital to the finished product here.

Colleen and Dell Hanks gave me the tools to be successful in life, encouraged me in this endeavor, and helped edit and review this book. Remember reviewing my first college essay, Mom? Hopefully this is some validation of your patient efforts over the years!

Thanks also to my in-laws Craig and Debbie Swensen who first introduced me to the dental world. That first invitation to a financial planning conference in Dallas has turned into a career. What a great gift!

Get Help!

I would love to work directly with you.

Get a FREE phone consultation about your specific situation or find out about working directly with me.

Email Me Directly:
Brian@BrianHanks.com

Or Visit **www.BrianHanks.com**

FOREWORD

Congratulations! You've made a very wise decision.

No, not picking up this book (Although that does prove you're insightful and highly intelligent!) Congratulations for choosing one of the best careers I know of: dentistry.

Congratulations on getting into college, into dental school, surviving dental school, and possibly a residency, and now wanting to own your own practice.

You've made so many good decisions already in life, you *should* feel good about where you are. Feel confident. You've made good choices. Working with folks like you all day, I know dentistry is an incredibly rewarding career choice. You get to master a craft where you're positively impacting people's health. You get to help them improve their smile and feel better about themselves. You have tons of flexibility in how you practice, plus you are paid well to do it all.

And now you've made the wise decision to buy a practice.

Congratulations.

Now, don't screw it all up.

What do I mean? I mean the stakes to buy the right practice for you are high. Get this step wrong and you're looking at stress, money worries, angry staff and patients, and a frustrated family that doesn't see you as much as they'd like.

On the other hand I've seen happy, fulfilled, relaxed, and wealthy dentists thriving in their career, positively impacting the lives of their patients, and living the life of their dreams. Many of the happy dentists own their practice, and they love being owners.

Thousands of dentists go through the process of buying a dental practice every year. Did they make a good decision on their practice? Did they buy at the right price? Did they buy at the right time?

The Pride Institute did a survey[1] of hundreds of buyers of dental practices. About 35% of buyers were first-timers, buying their first dental practice. 25% of buyers were relocating to another area, and 22% of buyers were acquiring another practice because they were trying to acquire more patients. The remainder were upgrading or preventing competition.

This book provides a step-by-step blueprint of the process of buying a dental practice that is right for you. I break the practice purchase process into five steps, including steps to take before and after you buy.

Step 1	Step 2	Step 3	Step 4	Step 5
Before You Buy	Find & Analyze a Practice	Due Diligence	Plan & Execute	First Steps as an Owner

A note to the two intended audiences of this book:

First-time buyers – Follow each of the five steps to confidently purchase a dental practice.

Veteran practice owners – Feel free to skip around the

---

[1] http://www.dentaleconomics.com/articles/print/volume-89/issue-10/features/to-buy-or-not-to-buy-your-move.html

steps to study the details that relate to wherever you find yourself in the purchase process.

Please know I've tried to be as helpful and accurate as possible throughout the book. You should, however, always confer with competent advisors before making major decisions. The specific advice and steps in this book will apply to 90% of buyers, 90% of the time. It's entirely possible you're the exception to the rule. Buying a dental practice is a huge decision and a complex process. Don't try to do it on your own. Use this book as the resource to help you know what to ask and what to expect, and then get competent help.

Let's dive in.

Step 1	Step 2	Step 3	Step 4	Step 5
Before You Buy	Find & Analyze a Practice	Due Diligence	Plan & Execute	First Steps as an Owner

- Be Sure You Want to Own
- What to Do About Student Loans
- Best Steps After Dental School

STEP 1:
BEFORE YOU BUY

Buying a dental practice could be one of the best decisions you ever make. Owning your practice can lead to independence, control over your destiny, and big rewards. However, there's no doubt running your own practice is both challenging and risky. Before you take on more debt and responsibility, it's important to fully understand what it takes to be a successful practice owner.

Remember when they taught you all you need to know about buying and owning your own practice in dental school?

I didn't think so.

In one survey only 7% of dentists felt their dental school adequately prepared them from a business standpoint to own their own practice. By comparison, 86.9% felt prepared clinically.

Just because you went to dental school doesn't mean you're ready to own your own practice.

Are You Sure You Want to Be an Owner?

Running a business and clinically diagnosing and treating dental work are two different skills. Pretend for a moment you're Shaquille O'Neal, preparing to make a comeback and play basketball with the Lakers. You head to tryouts, and instead of a basketball the coach hands you a bat, glove and baseball and says, "show us what you can do."

A lot of newer practice owners feel like they've invested an immense amount of time and energy on mastering their clinical skills, and then they buy a practice. And it's like someone handed them baseball gear at a basketball tryout.

There's no question the most valuable skills you'll have in your career are your clinical skills. Your ability to diagnose and treat dental patients is probably your most financially valuable skill.

The second most valuable skill you'll have in your career, however, is your ability to run a business. The two skills are very, very different.

Once you buy the practice, you'll be marketing your services, hiring and managing employees, fixing the operations of the practice to make sure things run smoothly, negotiating with suppliers, reading financial statements, and on and on.

And you'll be the boss of it all the day you own the practice.

The dentists who are most successful both in terms of money and overall happiness are those that think of themselves as business owners who happen to be dentists, instead of as dentists who happen to own a business.

The good news is you don't have to know or even be good at everything from day one. You can, and should, hire help for some of the key business functions that need to get done. The rewards of ownership are absolutely worth the risk. You'll have total control over the types of dentistry you do. You'll have total control over the patients you see. And because you're taking on more risk and more responsibility, you'll probably receive a bigger paycheck than if you stay an employee.

But you need to go into the project of buying your dental practice with your eyes open and with the mindset of a business owner.

Shouldn't I Pay Off My Student Loans First?

Before we go too far, let's talk about the elephant in most of the conversations I have with newer dentists in the industry. When I bring up buying a practice, the most common phrase I hear when speaking at dental schools and residency programs across the country is:

"I am really interested in owning my own dental practice, but I think I need to pay down my student loans before I buy one."

It's a common response. But it's not a wise one.

If you're coming out of dental school, you probably have a mountain of student loans. The average balance is $261,149 for dentists graduating in 2016[2]. It feels daunting.

---

[2] http://www.asdanet.org/debt.aspx

And it only feels worse if you did a residency program. I get it. Your natural inclination with that much student debt is to hold off on adding *even more* debt in the form of a practice loan.

If you know you want to eventually own a practice, waiting is probably a mistake.

Chances are, the quickest way for you to pay down your student loans is to own a good dental practice as soon as possible.

Recently, a client of mine came out of dental school with just under $300,000 in student loans. He's married, and has three kids. He worked for about eight months as an associate, and then shopped and found a good practice to buy. Two years after purchasing, he's whittled his student loan debt load down to about $80,000 and is on track to finish paying them off less than four years after dental school. Sound nice?

The fact is, the quickest way to pay down your student loans is to have the money to pay them down, and the quickest way to have the money is, typically, to own a good dental practice.

Let's look at a simple example that helps illustrate the point. Let's say you're a new dental grad a year or two out of dental school and you've got the hand speed and skills to do $800,000 a year in production. If you're an employee of a big chain, you're probably taking home 25% of production, or $200,000. Good for you. Your Mom is proud, and your non-dental friends will make you pay for dinner.

(Figure 1.1)

	Employee	Owner
Production	$800,000	
	x25%	
Your Salary	$200,000	

What if you were the same dentist, but instead were an owner?

As an owner, let's say you produce the same $800,000 in production and buy a practice producing exactly that amount per year. Let's assume you pay 65% of production for the practice, or $520,000. Now, instead of 25% of whatever you produce, you get to keep all the profits from the business. The average dental practice has overhead of about 60%, so you would get to keep about 40% as profit, or $320,000. But, don't forget you had to get a loan to buy the practice. Let's say it was a 10-year loan at a 5% interest rate. That's $66,185 annually you'd need to pay towards the loan. If you subtract the loan amount from the profit you have left from the business, you have $253,815 – $53,815 more than you would have as an employee.

(Figure 1.2)

	Employee	Owner
Production	$800,000	$800,000
Business Expenses		($580,000)
Debt (5% Loan)		($66,185)
Your Salary	$200,000	$253,815

The real kicker comes down the road. After you've paid off the practice loan, you're now keeping all the profit from the business. If you're an employee, you're still making 25% of production.

(Figure 1.3)

	Employee	Owner
Production	$800,000	$800,000
Business Expenses		($580,000)
Debt (5% Loan)		($66,185)
Your Salary	$200,000	$253,815
Your Salary in 10 Years	$200,000	$320,000

Of course, in real life the comparison is never quite as simple. There are other financial factors I haven't mentioned, and plenty of non-financial factors not included in this analysis. Do you want control over which procedures you recommend? Do you want control over whom you work with? Do you want the added stress that comes with owning a business? Answers to those questions matter as much as the numbers.

Even assuming ownership is still the goal, after I run students through the numbers I get this common objection: *"With as much as I have in student loans, no bank will lend to me! How can I get a loan?"*

Banks can and frequently do lend to newer dentists with large student loan balances. Banks love to lend to dentists. It's true you'll need to buy a dental practice that can support your student loan payments along with your living expenses at home. But make no mistake – the banks will run those numbers backwards and forwards. A good dental accountant can run the cash flow projections for you as well. I'd be willing to bet good money you *(and your student loans)* can get a practice loan. (Skip ahead to Chapter 3 for details on how to get a practice loan.)

If you have a general idea of the pros and cons of business ownership, and you suspect you will someday want to own your own practice, don't wait until your student loans are paid off. The fastest way to pay off those pesky student loans is to have the money to pay them off. And generally, the quickest way to have that money is to own a good dental practice sooner rather than later.

Your Best Steps Immediately After Dental School or Residency

If you have a business owner's mentality, and you're ready to pay down those student loans as an owner your best step right out of dental school is go out and immediately buy a practice, right?

Wrong.

If you're just graduating, you probably don't have the experience you need yet. You need to focus on two things:

First, improve your clinical skills & increase your hand speed. You need some day-in day-out time with patients to increase your speed and master your procedures. In baseball terminology, you need some at-bats. Make sure you're in a job (either as an employee or associate) where you'll be seeing a lot patients.

Second, work somewhere where you'll see exactly what it's like to be an owner. Work hard to find an associate job, or employment arrangement where you'll be at least partially compensated based on production or collections. If you know you want to be an owner someday, why would you search for any job other than one where you'll be focused on the same things you'll be focused on as an owner –

speed, diagnosis, case acceptance, marketing to new patients, etc.?

As a future owner, going to work for a corporate dental chain is probably among your worst options. Picking up bad habits is a hidden danger of working as an employee at a big corporate dental chain right out of school. As an employee you're more comfortable with an open schedule. You're slower than your colleagues who own their own practice. You aren't quite as good at selling the need for a procedure to your patient. Why would you be? The buck, ultimately, stops with someone else. I frequently see new practice owners who come from the corporate dental world struggle as owners.

I once helped a doctor transition from his job in a corporate dental chain to owning his own dental practice. By far the hardest part of the transition for him was the mentality shift of going from employee to owner. "When a patient cancelled at the last minute I used to cheer," he told me. "Now that I'm the owner, I can't afford to do that anymore. I feel like I'm always running full speed at work now."

Ideally, find a job as an associate in a practice of a similar size and demographic you eventually want to own. Yes, it would be great to work for a dentist who is a year or two away from retiring and then buy her practice. Go into that type of associateship knowing it probably won't work out. It's very hard to know exactly what you'll want in a practice immediately after dental school. (And those doctors that say they *want* to retire soon frequently find out they're not quite ready after two years for various reasons and tend to stick around longer than you'd like.)

Working as an associate in an office that is similar to the one you might eventually buy is the best course of action right out of dental school. You get the experience you need, pick up the best habits of a business owner, and get an idea of how you will run your practice when you own it.

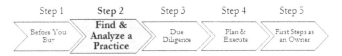

- How to Find a Practice
- Choose Your Team
- Practice Value & Analysis
- Cash Flow Analysis
- The Letter of Intent

STEP 2:
FIND AND ANALYZE A PRACTICE

A friend of mine builds custom homes and recently worked with clients building their dream home. The clients had a hard time deciding on a floor plan, but finally came to an agreement on what they wanted. The architect was called, plans were drawn up, and the project started. The foundation crew came to the lot and poured the cement.

Then the clients changed their minds. They wanted to change the size of some bedrooms, and the location of the kitchen. "Too late." My friend told them. "Once the foundation is poured, the number of changes you can make is very limited."

The dental practice you buy is the foundation of your career. Once you've purchased a practice, the number of changes you can make in your career is severely limited.

Once you buy a practice, where you live is fixed for a while, as well as how far from the practice it is practical to live. Several factors that contribute to your practice's success are largely outside your control, like patient demographics, insurance firms in your area, the number of competitors, and referral sources.

Buy the right practice and all of those factors can work toward your benefit and act like a tail wind to your success. That just makes finding the right practice much more important.

How to Find a Dental Practice to Buy

Finding the right practice to buy can be, for some, the most frustrating part of the entire practice purchase process.

But how to find the right practice? And what if you can't find the right practice quickly? Several of your friends from dental school had connections or family that helped them get started. Some of your other friends have mentors who have helped. But for whatever reason, you're coming up dry. Or you don't know where to start. What to do?

I work with a lot of dentists with tons of good options they're trying to decide amongst. I also work with a lot of dentists who struggle to find *anything* worthwhile to consider. What makes the difference? In my experience, there is one overriding principle followed by those who find lots of practice options to purchase – they have a broad, deep and friendly network in the dental community.

Most newer dentists are terrible at this. I know because when I ask them about their process to find a practice to buy, they have no network.

Notice I did NOT say the skill you need is "networking." I'm not talking about handing out your business cards at cocktail parties, schmoozing up a storm. Too many people, including me, don't like that kind of "networking."

I am suggesting you build and maintain a strong network amongst those who are in the dental community. Who should you focus on building your network with?

Other Dentists Are Your Best Source

By far the most effective networks I see that help dentists find practices to buy are networks of other dentists. You should talk to anyone who's a dentist and incorporate them into your network. Be indiscriminate. You're not looking for life-long friends or god-parents for your children. You're looking for knowledge about the marketplace and an inside track on opportunities in your target area.

Imagine yourself as a successful veteran of an area, and a new dental grad offers to take you to lunch to ask questions and gain some of your vast wisdom. You'd feel flattered! So will the dentists in the area where you're looking. Plus, they may know of a doctor (or themselves!) who are thinking about selling. A sharp, promising young dentist looking to buy could be just the nudge they need.

Dental Practice Transition Brokers

Most practices today are still sold through brokers. Find several practice transition brokers who work in the region of the country you're interested in and contact them. A simple Google search will work, for example: "dental practice transition brokers Houston." Don't forget to expand the geography of your web search beyond just a city to a state or region. And there's no reason why you can't be working with several brokers at a time.

Even if these brokers don't have a practice listed that interests you, I still recommend you contact them and get on their mailing list for future opportunities. Remember brokers get paid by the seller. As friendly and as effective as many of them are, they ultimately work for the seller. Brokers will want you in their network, too, but mostly because they hope to sell you a practice someday.

Dental Supply/Equipment Reps

If you know the state and city you want to live in, dental equipment reps can be a great resource. Call around and ask who the Patterson/Schein/Burkhart reps are and then call them directly. These folks have their ear to the ground and regularly talk with a lot of dentists in your target area. Take them to coffee and ask for their opinion on the area, demographics, different PPO providers, etc. They know a lot, and you could be one of their next clients. Show them you're serious about buying, and they may know of opportunities for sale before anyone else.

Dental Society Websites

I've had several clients find practices on the classified section for state and city dental associations that weren't listed elsewhere. Some dentists are interested in selling their practice themselves before involving brokers, and you just may find something here you wouldn't find other places.

If you're in the process of looking for a practice and are having trouble finding one, you likely have one of two problems. First, the area you're searching in may be too small. If you're from a small town and want to move back home, you might need to wait for a practice to come on the market.

The second (and frankly more likely) reason you can't find a practice to buy is that your personal network isn't as strong as it needs to be. The best time to start building your network was yesterday. The second-best time to start is today, so jump in.

The most important point to remember is to cast your net wide. Don't just work with one broker. Don't just look at one practice. Keep your options open, and talk to everyone!

When you think you've found the practice of your dreams, keep your eyes open. I've seen many young doctors put all their eggs in one seller's basket, only to have the seller sell to someone else at the last minute. Keep your network wide, deep, and active until you've closed on your practice.

Assembling Your Team

One of the most successful baseball players of the last generation, Derek Jeter, was popular not only for his success on the field but for his reputation as a genuinely good person. He said:

"Surround yourself with good people. People who are going to be honest with you and look out for your best interests."

Jeter's advice is just as applicable to dentists as it is to the major leagues. You shouldn't expect to learn everything you need to know to correctly navigate the practice purchasing waters. I strongly recommend surrounding yourself with good, professional, competent, and ethical advisors both for the process of purchasing your practice, as well as the ongoing financial management of your business.

But how do you decide who will meet all those criteria? How do you know who is truly looking out for you?

As you're getting advice on all the aspects of buying a dental practice it's important to get advice from people "on the team" as I like to call it. People on the team are those who have both the experience and knowledge you need, and your best interests in mind when giving advice.

In the accounting and finance world where I work there is a term to describe those who have your best interests in mind when providing advice: Fiduciary. A fiduciary is one who gives you the same advice they would give themselves if they were in your shoes. A fiduciary should provide complete honesty in the advice they provide you earning total trust and good faith.

Your mom is probably an example of a person who gives you advice with no hidden agenda. She gave birth to you, changed your diapers, and is probably going to give you advice with nothing but your best interests in mind. Moms are the best. The problem with mom giving you advice on your dental practice purchase is she doesn't have a lot of experience dealing with dental transitions. (Unless she's a dentist, of course! If that's the case for you, just do whatever mom tells you to do.)

By contrast, you'll talk with brokers, equipment reps, accountants, lawyers, other dentists, and many, many other people who DO have some experience with dental transitions. And they're generally not shy about giving you advice and telling you what your best option is. How do you know if those people have your best interests in mind?

My rule is simple:

The only advisors truly on your team when buying a practice, are those you pay directly.

(Figure 2.1)

On the Team	Not on the Team
Dental Accountant	Banker
Paid Directly by you. No commissions. Held to a Fiduciary standard. Advice given should be free from	Commission based on loan amount.
	Broker
	Paid by seller when practice sold.
Dental Attorney	Insurance Agent
Paid Directly by you. No commissions. Regulated by state bar association to protect your interests.	Commission on insurance amount.
	Equipment Rep
	Commission on equipment sold.
	Consultants
	Helpful after the transition.

Choosing your team is all about aligning incentives. Other players are key to you owning a practice. The only people really *on* your team with incentives aligned as closely as possible to yours, are your accountant and attorney.

You should directly pay both. Your dental accountant will help you understand the financial implications of one of the largest financial decisions of your life. Your attorney will protect you from a legal standpoint.

Your accountant and attorney should specialize in working with dentists. As a dentist, you know the value of specialization. The entire dental field is based on funneling the right cases to the right doctor for the job. The same principle applies here. Every dentist buying a dental practice should use an experienced accountant and attorney, both who specialize in helping dentists buying a dental practice.

Before I lay out how to choose and what to expect from your dental accountant and attorney, a quick note about the other folks involved in your transition: You absolutely need a good banker, broker, insurance rep, and equipment rep to assist through the transition. They will be crucial in completing the purchase of your practice. Take the time to carefully decide between several of those folks who you enjoy working with and who you'll pay. However, recognize even the best bankers, brokers, and insurance and equipment reps have some bias built into the advice they're providing and adjust your actions accordingly.

How to Choose Your Dental Accountant

Your dental accountant's job is to analyze the economic side of the deal and how it will impact your personal finances. Look for someone with experience with dental transitions. Ask if they receive any referral fees from brokers or banks ("No." is the correct answer.)

The fee to engage a dental accountant through the deal will typically range anywhere from $4,500 to $12,000. Some dental accountants will charge a small retainer, with the balance due upon completion of the deal and the bank loan funding. A good dental accountant will help you answer these three key questions:

1. Is this a good practice to buy?
2. If yes, what is a fair price to pay for this practice?
3. If I pay that much, how much can I expect to make as owner?

Choosing your accountant is one of the most important decisions you make when you buy a dental practice. You don't want to get it wrong. A good dental accountant will help you understand the financial implications of any dental practice you're considering, including purchase price, tax impacts, and how much money you might make after you're an owner.

Good dental accountants will not only help you run numbers and provide analysis, they'll help get you financially set up to be an owner. Many can, and do, assist you with the items on your "buyer's checklist" (see Chapter 3)—financial due diligence, IRS forms filings, insurance reviews, accounting and banking setup, etc.

When considering the purchase of a dental practice, interview two or three dental accountants and ask the following questions:

1. Do you specialize in working with dental practice transitions and dental practice owners?
2. How many clients do you work with? How many are you working with now?
3. What are some of the basic philosophical principles that drive your recommendations to clients?
4. What services do you provide?
5. How will you help set me up for success when I'm an owner?
6. Can I speak with some existing and previous clients as a referral?
7. How much do you charge and when do you charge it?
8. How often will we be speaking through the transition? How will we coordinate meetings?

How to Choose Your Dental Attorney

Your attorney's job is to protect you legally and help negotiate a good deal overall. You want an attorney with experience in dental transitions. Most attorneys aren't limited by geography when doing these types of transactions, but ask your attorney about any state-specific laws that may apply. The fee to engage a dental attorney through the deal will typically range anywhere from $4,000 to $15,000. Some attorneys will charge a flat fee, while others charge an hourly rate. Personally, I like the flat fee option for most of the clients I work with. An attorney working on a flat fee basis has fewer incentives to work more hours just to increase a bill. Similarly, you'll be less worried about reaching out with questions when you know those questions won't increase the bill. A good dental attorney will help you with several very important steps, including:

1. Review and negotiate the Letter of Intent
2. Review and negotiate terms of the practice purchase contract.
3. Review and negotiate terms of the lease or building purchase.
4. Help set up a business entity.

Carefully choosing a good dental attorney is a crucial step when buying a dental practice. A good attorney understands how to buy a dental practice and can literally save you hundreds of hours of stress and hundreds of thousands of dollars.

Many dental practice buyers choose to save money and rely on the seller's lawyer. This is a huge mistake.

Some dentists choose to use a lawyer they know personally, but who lacks experience to represent them in one of the most important (and costly!) career decisions of their life. Another huge mistake.

I once worked with a recent dental school grad buying a dental practice in Georgia. He got a recommendation for a local attorney who was competent, but didn't specialize in dental transitions. The attorney didn't know about warranties on dental work and the buyer had to re-do some very costly crown work the seller should have at least partially covered. This one omission cost the new dentist close to $20,000 in his first three months of business.

The worst part was when the buyer received the lawyer's bill, it was based on an hourly rate. The bill was three to four times higher than a flat-rate dental attorney would have charged. Another $10,000+ expenditure in the first few months of business!

What Does a Lawyer Do When You're Buying a Dental Practice?

Your lawyer should be involved in at least four key areas of your dental practice purchase: reviewing the Letter of Intent, creating or reviewing the Purchase Agreement, renewing and negotiating the lease, and creating the right entity for your practice.

Reviewing the Letter of Intent

The Letter of Intent (LOI) is the document you negotiate with the seller around the major terms of the deal – price, timing, etc. It is a document that is typically legally non-binding—essentially a piece of paper both the buyer and seller sign saying, "we want the transition to look like this…"

Some brokers will discourage getting a lawyer involved in the transition at this stage "to save money." This is a bad idea for you as the buyer. Typically, the broker wants you to feel locked into what is in the letter of intent before you hire competent advisors. Both your attorney or accountant can help with the negotiations at this crucial stage of discussions with the seller.

A properly negotiated LOI can literally save you hundreds of thousands of dollars, protect both you and the seller, and increase the chance your purchase will be successful. (see Chapter 3 on what your LOI should include.)

Creating or Reviewing the Purchase Agreement

The purchase agreement is the document that ultimately transfers ownership of the dental practice. Having an attorney you pay to negotiate and help review this document is absolutely crucial.

You want to see an agreement that protects you from the seller competing with you post-sale. You want an agreement that deals with accounts receivable and uncompleted work, not to mention protecting you regarding warranty issues of the seller's patients coming back in with problems you didn't cause, but need to fix "for free." The purchase agreement will deal with patient retention, employee benefits, the asset allocation, tax treatment of goodwill, and several other important issues.

Everyone believes their transition will be smooth and they have a great relationship with their new best friend, the seller. The reality is that transitions sometimes go bad. One of the best ways to prevent that from happening is to have a well-written purchase agreement both parties understand and agree to.

Reviewing and Negotiating the Lease

Your lease is one of the most expensive monthly bills you'll have as an owner of a dental practice. And unlike dental supplies or lab fees, once the ink is dry on the lease, you don't have the ability to lower your monthly lease cost for sometimes a decade or more.

It's crucial to have an attorney review your lease to ensure the core issues in the lease are fair and protect both parties. You're more likely to get rent modified or get additional lease periods with the help of an attorney with experience negotiating dental spaces. This review could save you tens or even hundreds of thousands of dollars over the life of your lease.

Your dental attorney reads every word of the lease, unlike a broker or agent. The dental attorney is looking for smaller things, like who owns the trade fixtures and what constitutes a default. The goal of your dental attorney should be to ensure there isn't some obscure provision in any of your sale documents that could cause you a headache.

I'll include a little information on buying the building, however I won't cover the topic in great detail here. Whether or not you buy the building depends on too many factors to give a blanket recommendation. I tell my clients that they can spend a lot of money renting their building, or they can spend a lot of money owning the building. One recommendation I can give with a measure of confidence is to check your assumptions about real estate before assuming that buying the building is automatically the best option. Often purchasing the building is more headaches than new owners realize. Another recommendation that generally holds true is to split the timing of purchasing the practice and building, if possible. I've seen so many deals get sidelined for weeks and even months around some issue or another related to the building, when everything on the practice purchase side is ready to go. This won't always be possible, but it's a good rule of thumb.

Whether or not you buy the building will depend on your geography, specific situation, lending options, and appetite for landlord responsibilities. Work closely with legal, accounting and real estate professionals before choosing to buy the building.

Creating the Right Entity for Your Practice

How do you know whether you should be an S-corporation, LLC, or sole proprietorship when buying your dental practice? A good dental transitions lawyer can help you know both the legal and monetary impacts of the most common choices. Combine the lawyer's advice with your dental accountant's, and you can protect yourself, and your business, and minimize the taxes you'll pay as an owner.

Your state will have rules around what types of entities you can choose as a dental practice and what names you are allowed to use. A good dental transitions attorney can help you choose the right entity for your practice. Additionally, they will be the ones to file the documents with your state to open the entity and get you a legal business.

Dental attorneys should also help with the naming of your business. They'll do a search to see if your name is available, and what other names will be similar in your area possibly causing patient confusion. Depending on your state, they might trademark your name or help you with a DBA ("doing business as") and explain why that could benefit your new practice.

Buying a dental practice is one of the most important decisions a dentist makes in their career. The decisions you make throughout the process of buying a dental practice are complex and unique to the dental profession. Using a dental-transition-specific lawyer is the best way to ensure all your bases are covered. It will cost you some money in the short-term, but the right lawyer can ultimately save you tens and even hundreds of thousands of dollars over your career.

> Need a recommendation of a good dental attorney? I know several around the country that do excellent work for their dental transition clients. Contact me via email **Brian@BrianHanks.com** for qualified referrals because a good attorney can protect you and your investment of time and money.

Conflicts of Interest for Accountants & Attorneys

Did you know dental accountants and attorneys often receive offers to sell you out and refer products and services that might not be the best for you?

I received the email below in 2016 from a web marketer who wanted to show me his amazing search engine optimization (SEO) and traffic driving skills. His ultimate goal is to get me to refer my clients over to him. Watch how he phrases the offer:

"…I also wanted to reach out to see if any of your dental clients have any interest in a digital marketing campaign. I have been working with "[Dr. Jones]" for years now, and his SEO campaign has consistently brought new patients to his practice. If you're able to connect me with any of your clients who want my support, I'd love to discuss a Finder's Fee relationship with you for making the connection."

A "finder's fee relationship?" That's a polite way to say he'll pay me for referrals.

There's some good news and some bad news here. First, the bad news:

Because you (presumably) have a trusting relationship with your accountant and attorney, those folks get offers like this often. I receive a few of these every year. Other accounting firms get them and, unfortunately, don't turn them down. It's so common, frequently the service providers who offer these referral arrangements are shocked when I tell them to take a hike. There must be a lot of accountants out there who augment their income with these kickbacks!

Here is an example of how it works during a dental transition: A client needs a loan to buy a dental practice. The client asks her accountant for advice on whom to work with. The accountant says "You have to work with so-and-so bank. They have the best rates right now!" Meanwhile, the accountant and the banker involved haven't disclosed the referral fee that gets paid as a result of the introduction. The client never shops around, not knowing a better loan was just a few phone calls away, and is worse off financially as a result.

It's not just bankers who provide "referral fees" either. Dental consultants, 401k providers, mutual fund companies, etc. The list of potential conflicts of interest is long.

Fortunately, there is some good news. The first piece of good news is you are now armed with knowledge, and you know to ask the question, "do you have a financial relationship with this firm you're recommending?" My advice is to always ask the question. The answer should be "no" or you should feel very comfortable with the disclosure that is made.

The second piece of good news is there are honest, ethical dental accountants and attorneys out there who will always put your interests first, turning down these referral fees. Ask the question and choose to work with one of those firms.

What You Need to Know About Everyone Else

A deal can't come together with just an accountant and lawyer. The rest of the folks below are crucial to buying a practice. Usually, they'll have good advice you should consider. Why are they not "on the team?" Because at some level their incentives are not perfectly aligned with yours. Almost everyone has the best of intentions, but ignoring the incentives of the person giving you advice on one of the largest financial transactions of your life is just foolish.

Consider the following as you work with other players on your deal:

Banker

A good banker is worth his weight in gold. He'll provide valuable advice and help you avoid pitfalls. If he's so important, why is he not 'on the team?' Simple. Bankers are incentivized by loan amount. The more you borrow, the better for them. Borrowing more is not always necessarily best for you.

Broker

Good brokers are incredibly important, too. Just like bankers, brokers work on deals 24/7 so they typically know the good practices from the bad. However, brokers are paid by the seller, so any grey area on a deal will naturally bias a broker towards the seller. Beyond the purchase price you'll need to work out the tax implications of the asset allocation, whether or not to purchase the accounts receivable and at what price, and other details. A good broker will work hard to get his or her client (the seller) the best terms for those elements of the deal. You should care a great deal about those deal points. A higher purchase price and a quick close are the top concerns of brokers, but may not be yours.

Equipment Rep

An equipment rep you like and trust will be important as an owner, even after the purchase. Additionally, during the transition he can provide a perspective on the value and usefulness of the equipment of the practice you're buying. However, equipment reps make money when you buy equipment. You may or may not need new equipment now while buying the practice.

Insurance Agent

You'll have all kinds of insurance policies as a practice owner. A good insurance agent will help protect you from catastrophe, while not overpaying for insurance you don't need. Just like bankers may have an incentive to oversell, insurance agents get paid when you buy lots of insurance. The misalignment of incentives is therefore something to be aware of.

Practice Management & Marketing Consultants

Hiring a consultant to help can be extremely valuable. However, your top priority when buying a practice is cash flow. Consultants cost money. Look at a practice and/or marketing consultant after you've been an owner for a little while.

How Dental Practice Valuations Work

Some dentists think there is a "right" price for every dental practice on the market. They assume dental practices are like home values, where someone out there with the right formula can input some numbers into a calculator and get the "fair appraised" value for any practice available. The appraisal is therefore the gospel truth. These dentists know, just like buying a house, the two parties might haggle a bit over the sales price, but the anchor point of the negotiation is the appraisal.

In reality, valuing a business, including a dental practice, is a much more subjective process than most dentists realize.

Let me share how valuations work in reality with a quick story from my MBA program.

I learned how business valuations work in one of the most difficult finance classes I've ever taken. Week in and week out our professor drilled us in the various methods of valuing a business—discounted cash flow, multiples method, comparable transactions, market valuation, sum of parts method, etc. We showed up each week with our models, and had them mercilessly torn apart by the professor. He had to be tough! He was training the next generation of Wall Street bankers. But I was learning the "right" way to value a business. On the last day of class, I learned all that work would be put to a different use than I expected.

Our professor ended the semester by saying, "Every

valuation you do outside of class will be complete bull. To get hired by a client to even do the valuation in the first place, you'll need to sell them the *story* that you can get a buyer to pay *more* than any of the other brokers out there. You're going to tell the client a number of how much their business is worth, and then you're going to back into that number by choosing the model and assumptions that get you the number the client wanted to see in the first place. And the client will only be happy if they get *that* number."

He was saying the valuation is completely made up!

Dental brokers are no different when they do valuations. If you've seen a valuation number for a dental practice, it is a series of assumptions piled on imperfect information. The seller hired that broker, in part, because the broker convinced them they could get them the most for their dental practice. Oh sure, the number needs to be believable. It can't be totally crazy and needs to fall within an acceptable range. But the formula isn't as precise as some dental buyers assume.

So how do you know what a dental practice is *really* worth? Technically, the only way to know for sure what a practice is worth is to find a number where a willing buyer will pay to a willing seller. Once you and a seller agree on the price, you've found the "right" value for the practice.

That said, you don't want to be ripped off. The two methods I use to see if clients are paying a fair price are:

1. Price to Gross Revenue
2. Price to Earnings

I'll explain what these methods mean, and how to think about them.

Price to Gross Revenue

This method describes how much you need to pay for the collections of a dental practice. This is the method most people are familiar with. It basically says, "how much will I pay for a dollar of collections?" The historical average of that number is the average buyer pays the average seller is 69.87% or $0.70 (rounded up) for $1.00 of collections. Put differently, if a practice collects $1,000,000, then it sells for about $698,700.

Price to Earnings

This method describes how much you need to pay for the earnings of a dental practice. It says, "how much will I pay for a dollar of net income from the practice after all the expenses are paid." Earnings are how much the practice has left over after expenses, but before any pay and perks of the doctor. The historical average here says buyers pay about $1.61 for $1.00 of earnings. Put differently, if a practice has annual earnings of exactly $100,000, the average buyer in the US will pay $161,000.

Which Method is Better?

You should put significantly *more* weight on the Price to Earnings method. I care more about how much money I'm keeping after all my work than I do about how much the practice collects. True, you want to know *both* numbers to know if you're getting a good deal on your dental practice. Let me explain what I mean with a few visual examples. Let's say you are looking at this dental practice below.

(Figure 2.2)

Dental Practice A

	Income
Collections	$1,000,000
	Expenses
Salary & Benefits	$300,000
Dental Supplies	$60,000
Lab Fees	$60,000
Office Expenses	$20,000
Rent	$50,000
Everything Else	$110,000
Total Expenses	$600,000
PROFIT	$400,000

Simple Dental Practice A is a typical practice, where I used average data and simple round numbers to show a practice that collects $1 Million, has expenses totaling $600,000 and profit left over for the doctor of $400,000. (Indeed, the average dental practice has overhead totaling about 60% of collections.)

Simple Dental Practice B is exactly the same in every way, but this doctor pays her staff **much** better. Higher pay, maybe she pays for health insurance and a pension of some variety. There's probably a few extra staff members around, too. (You wouldn't want people to work too hard, right?)

(Figure 2.3)

Dental Practice B

	Income
Collections	$1,000,000
	Expenses
Salary & Benefits	$500,000
Dental Supplies	$60,000
Lab Fees	$60,000
Office Expenses	$20,000
Rent	$50,000
Everything Else	$110,000
Total Expenses	$800,000
PROFIT	$200,000

Now, let's say you're considering buying these two practices. Which would you rather buy? And which one should be cheaper?

Easy answer, right? You'd want Practice A, because as the owner there is more profit left over for you at the end of the year.

In reality *both practices will be valued at about the same amount by most valuation models*. I swear I'm not lying. This is exactly what most brokers do. Oh sure, I just ticked off every broker I know, and their valuations always look a lot fancier with big long spreadsheets on how they arrived at their number. But, with an uncanny degree of accuracy, if I only know collections numbers, I can tell you within about 3% what any given broker valued a practice.

Given you're buying a business, and you're going to live off the profit of the business, wouldn't you rather put more weight on the Price to Earnings method? Wouldn't you rather buy Practice A, instead of Practice B, all other things being equal?

Of course you would.

But, here's the rub, *all other things never are equal.* And every seller can give you a list of 100 reasons why you should still pay top dollar, even though they're not as profitable as they could be.

While my goal with practice valuation analysis is to help a buyer pay a fair price for a practice, I frequently will help buyers keep the big picture in perspective. Remember you don't make most of your money buying and selling dental practices. Oh sure, you definitely don't want to overpay when buying a dental practice. But, the real money in dentistry comes in the year-in, year-out ownership of the profit stream from the business.

If they've found a good practice that isn't as profitable as it could be, I tell my clients to think about the profit stream of the business as the primary consideration. Use the Price to Earnings methodology to negotiate and bring the seller down a bit on price, if necessary. But, if you like the city the practice is in, your spouse likes the area, the building is good, the staff seems good, the equipment isn't junk and you think you can make it work . . . don't get hung up on which valuation method you use to value the practice.

Don't overpay, but don't make the mistake that you can mathematically figure out the value of a dental practice.

Average Dental Practice Values

What are some benchmarks you can use to know if the dental practice you're considering purchasing is priced fairly?

For buyers, specifically, the answer to this question is the second of the three big questions when buying a dental practice:

1) Is this a good practice to buy?
2) If yes, what price is fair to pay?
3) If I pay that much, how much should I expect to make?

The table below can be helpful to orient yourself around a typical Price to Collections valuation of a practice you're looking at.

(Figure 2.4)

Specialty	Average Price to Collections	Number of Transactions
General Dentistry	69.87%	428
Orthodontics	79.81%	202
Oral Surgery	68.57%	53
Pediatric Dentistry	71.22%	69
Periodontics	65.62%	39
Endodontics	67.61%	15
Prosthodontics	67.13%	9

¹ 15 Year Period beginning Jan '01

Average fair market value to collections looks at the sales price relative to the amount of annual revenue, usually over the last one to three years. For example, if an oral surgery practice collecting $1,000,000 sold for an average of 68.57%, the sales price would be $685,700.

The most valuable type of dental practice continues to be orthodontics at 79.81% of collections. Pediatric dental practices as second most valuable at 71.22%.

General dental practices are the next most valuable, currently selling for an average of 69.87% of annual collections, followed by oral surgery at 68.57%.

Endodontics practices are slightly lower at 67.61% and periodontics practices command the lowest prices at 65.62%. It's important to note prosthodontics practices are on the lower end of the spectrum at 67.13%, but the volume is low enough not to cross the line of a statistically significant sample size. The true average value could be lower or higher, and without more data I can't state for sure which is the case. If I'm buying or selling a prosthodontics practice, I would note that average practice values are on the lower end, but more likely reflect the average overall dental transitions market.

It's important to remember that fair market value to collections, while the most common valuation method, is not the only method to value a practice. Similar data using the Price to Earning method is unfortunately not available.

As this book is written in 2017 practice values are going up, in general, across the country. Several factors contribute to the rising prices. The most fundamental is the basic market dynamic of supply and demand. Dentists are working longer with the average retiring age closer to 70 than 65 (because they choose to, or because they didn't have good financial advice along the way!) Fewer retiring dentists means a lower supply of established practices for sale, increasing prices.

Another key factor is a dramatic rise in the number of corporate buyers in the market. Profit margins are so high in dentistry, relative to other industries, that venture capital and private equity funds are looking to get in on the action. This brings even more demand for the fewer dental practices for sale!

Newer dentists looking to buy are facing the double-whammy of fewer dental practices generally available, and more buyers looking to buy them. When they find a practice for sale and ask, "how much is this dental practice worth?" the answer is probably, "more than it was five years ago."

The Good News About Dental Practice Values

While the *trends* in dental practice values are going up, without question buyers *should* continue to look at purchasing a practice as a solid career strategy. Again, while no one wants to overpay for their dental practice, the clear fact is that ownership of the income stream of a dental practice continues to be the most financially lucrative career choice in dentistry.

Another key fact in the buyers' corner is that bank lending is readily available today. More and more banks understand dental transitions and are getting in the game. All the reputable dental lenders will fund 100% of the purchase price on a profitable dental practice with some basic caveats. Many lenders will lend *more* than 100% when a working capital loan is included in the picture.

While it is important to understand the trends, dental practices continue to be valuable for both buyers and sellers. As a buyer, know that you're going to pay a little bit more for your practice than you would have a few years ago. But the income stream produced from ownership of a *good* practice is still worth *every penny* you'll pay. With more buyers in the marketplace, it's more important than ever to work with a reputable dental attorney and accountant to help you move quickly through the process.

How to Evaluate a Practice

When I'm helping a dentist evaluate whether or not to put an offer on a practice I mentally split the decision into two bodies of analysis: the quantitative and the qualitative.

The quantitative is fairly straightforward. The numbers of the practice can help you answer questions about how much the practice is worth, how well it is run, and how much money you might make as the owner.

The qualitative side is less numerical, but no less important. The geography and physical location of your practice matter a great deal. Whether you like the area, have ties or family close by, and a thousand other non-financial factors can be either a head wind or tail wind in your success as a practice owner.

I'll cover both the quantitative and qualitative aspects of practice analysis and give you tools and questions to ask along the way in your own practice.

How to Analyze the Quantitative Factors

You can look at six or seven numbers in a practice you're considering buying and know, roughly speaking, a rough range of what the practice is worth and if it's worth buying. Step one, of course, is to look at the asking price and total collections and compare to the average values in the previous section of this book.

What about the rest of the numbers?

I'll outline exactly what to look for in a practice you're considering purchasing.

Key Number #1 – Collections

The foundation of whether to purchase any practice has to be collections. There simply must be enough money coming into the practice to justify the time, stress, and incredible expense you're going to take on as the owner of a practice. I recommend clients look at practices that have a minimum collections level of $800,000 a year; over $1 Million is even better. I've found, while not an iron-clad rule, practices collecting more than a million dollars annually tend to have good systems, solid staff, good locations, and all the foundational pieces you want as a business owner. On top of being well run, the projected cash flow numbers in practices that size tend to provide enough income to cover the practice loans, student loans and the desired lifestyle of newer dentists. Could you find a turnaround practice that has been mismanaged for years, buy it at a cheap price and turn it around? Possibly, but unlikely. More likely, the cheap practice you're looking at is struggling for a reason, and the reason isn't that the owner isn't as smart as you. That does mean you'll be excluding roughly 60-70% of the dental practices on the market from your search (see table 2.5).

(Figure 2.5)

Production Per Dentist for Private Practice Owners, 2015

	1st quartile	Median	3rd quartile	Standard deviation	Number of responses
General Practitioners					
All owners	$350,000	$575,000	$900,000	$387,550	672
Solo	$350,000	$600,000	$925,000	$400,060	458
Nonsolo	$337,500	$533,330	$800,000	$356,760	214
Specialists					
All owners	$566,000	$975,000	$1,333,330	$616,900	337
Solo	$600,000	$1,000,000	$1,319,820	$601,110	219
Nonsolo	$503,030	$905,000	$1,333,330	$646,260	118

Source: American Dental Association, Health Policy Institute, 2016 Survey of Dental Practice.

Key Number #2 – Profit

Deciding whether to buy, or the right price to pay for a practice doesn't depend on collections alone; you should also consider the overall profitability of the practice. The profit margin of the dental practice you're considering should be at least 40%. A 40% profit margin (or 60% overhead) is close to the average profitability of dental practices in the US. If the practice you're looking at is below that number, it could be a sign the practice isn't as well run as it should be. The staff might be overpaid. The systems to order supplies and work with labs might need a lot of work. The rent and other location-based expenses might be so high, you'll never make the kind of profit you might elsewhere.

Be careful here, though. The right profitability number is hard to know without some help.

How you calculate the profit number is more difficult than just looking at the "net income" number on the seller's profit and loss statement. To see the *true* profitability of a practice, you need to remove any "doctor-specific" expenses from the business. That includes the selling doctor's salary and associated payroll taxes. You need to back out any doctor perks, like meals and auto expenses, and interest, depreciation and amortization numbers. This is one service a good dental accountant that works with dental practice buyers should provide.

Bottom line: if profitability is strong and at least 40%, you probably are looking at a solid practice.

(Figure 2.6)

Median Annual Net Income of Dentists in Private Practice, 1990 – 2015

	1990	2000	2010	2015
General Practitioners				
All owners	$80,000	$141,660	$180,000	$172,000
Solo	$78,000	$129,000	$170,000	$150,000
Nonsolo	$90,000	$160,650	$200,000	$200,000
Employed	$40,000	$75,500	$110,000	$121,000
Specialists				
All owners	$125,000	$220,000	$254,000	$300,000
Solo	$115,000	$200,000	$216,000	$250,000
Nonsolo	$140,000	$254,450	$325,000	$367,000
Employed	--*	--*	$170,000	--*

Source: American Dental Association, Health Policy Institute, Surveys of Dental Practice.

* Too few observations for reliable statistical analysis.

Key Number #3 – Employee Expense Ratio

The largest expense in most dental practices is the staff. A well-run dental practice will typically have employee expenses range from 24% to 28% of collections. That includes salary, payroll taxes, and any employee benefits. You would think paying employees *more* would be better, right? Happier employees equal better employees and thus happier patients, right? Not quite. Remember we're talking about the ratio of employee pay to collections. The more you grow the practice, the more you can pay your employees, but the numbers should still be a reasonable percentage of overall collections.

Recently, I helped a buyer analyze a business for sale in the Northeast United States. The seller collected almost $1 Million a year, 38% of which was going towards employee expenses. I asked him about his approach. He stated "I just want my employees to be happy." They should have been. Each had an average of four vacation weeks a year, full 401k matching and profit share, and employer-paid health insurance. They were some of the best-paid dental employees on the planet. I wasn't shocked to see the practice was run about as well as the *average* practice I look at with buyers. The marketing was about average. Dental supplies expense (something the employees of this practice had direct control over) were actually a little higher than the average practice. The recall and treatment rates were only slightly above average.

Employees paid well over average didn't translate into an above-average practice. In this case, the only affect it had on the practice was a group of employees who felt entitled. On the plus side, turnover was low!

Furthermore, I learned many of these benefits had been added in the last ten years of the seller's tenure. The seller admitted they were overpaid, but didn't want to deal with the hassle of unhappy staff or turnover if he turned off the spigot to the gravy train. Instead he was hoping to pass the buck to the buyer of his practice. The buyer passed on the deal.

Key Number #4 – Lab Fees & Dental Supplies Ratio

Look for a practice that has a combined ratio of total lab fees and dental supplies expense in the range of 10% to 14%.

Of course, this number will differ slightly based on the type of practice. Orthodontists will spend more on supplies, and pediatric dentists less on lab fees. I find practices spending about 10% to 14% of their collections income on these two categories are careful about how they spend their money. This is the real secret of this number: While most large expenses like rent and employee expenses in a dental practice are relatively fixed (at least in the short term), lab fees and dental supplies are totally variable. They can be different every month and can be managed accordingly. If you see a practice with a low lab fee and dental supply ratio, chances are the owner of this practice is also managing other aspects of the business well.

Key Number #5 – Rent

There is no specific number to help use as a benchmark with rent. Real estate prices and costs are too local to be very specific here. However, there is a general principle to keep in mind: rent is a fixed cost not easily changed. If the rent number is high, changing that number downward is nearly impossible. Make sure the location you're considering actually matters to the patients who come to the office, and avoid locations built solely to help the selling doctor feel important.

Key Number #6 – Hours of Operation

This information isn't on the Profit and Loss statement, but is vital to know. Assuming the practice you're looking at is open Monday-Thursday, 8:00am-5:00pm when the hours are actually different could lead you to make mistakes in your analysis. In comparing two practices with similar collections and expense numbers, choosing the office with fewer open hours provides more opportunity for growth, or simply a better quality of life.

Key Number #7 – Will the Cash Flow Support My Goals?

So, I cheated a little to have this one in here, because this is more of an *analysis* and not one specific number. If the numbers of the practice you're considering purchasing work to this point, you'll want your dental accountant's help to project the cash flow from the business given your personal expenses. Of course, you'll add in your monthly student loan payments (if applicable) and how much you spend a month at home. Don't forget to include disability and life insurance payments, as well as savings and debt pay-down goals you've set for yourself.

When meeting with clients looking to buy a practice, I always show them the monthly and annual income they can have, assuming a seven-year practice loan payoff, as well as Roth IRA and 401k savings, in addition to potential changes they want to make with the practice. If the cash flow projections work, I always feel more comfortable with them moving forward with an offer on a good practice.

A quick recap is in order: to maximize your chances of purchasing a successful dental practice, make sure the practice you're considering purchasing meets the following basic criteria:

- Collections above $800,000.
- Profit Margins around 40% after backing out doctor-specific expenses.
- Employee expense ratio in the 24-28% range.
- Lab fees and dental supplies ratio in the 10-14% range (with some differences for different specialties).
- Rent isn't unreasonable, and you're not inheriting another doctor's Taj Mahal.
- Hours of operation fit the lifestyle or growth goals you've set for yourself.
- Cash flow projections allow enough money for savings, debt pay down and your lifestyle.

I can't emphasize enough the value of professional help in dealing with this decision. A good dental accountant who specializes in practice transitions will know all of the above and more. What's more, they will correctly help you in identifying and providing commentary on all the above categories for any practice you're considering. Just like an x-ray can almost talk to *you* as a dentist, a review of a practice's P&L and tax return are just like having the numbers sit up and tell a story. The story they tell can mean a good practice and smooth transition, or a bad practice and lots of heartache down the road.

> Need to talk with someone about the financial factors of a practice you're considering buying? I am happy to help you. Schedule a free consultation at **www.BrianHanks.com/connect** because an experienced eye can provide valuable insights.

How to Analyze the Qualitative Factors

Have you ever had a friend who wanted so badly to be in a relationship they talked themselves into being with someone who was a horrible match for them? Don't do the same thing with one of the largest purchasing decisions you'll ever make.

Buying a dental practice is a lot like finding someone to be in a serious relationship with. It's a huge decision. It's vitally important to get it right. And the consequences of choosing well or poorly will impact the quality of your life.

You've got to get the analysis right and for a dental practice, that means getting the numbers right. But it also means getting the qualitative factors right.

When looking for a practice to buy, it's obvious to an outsider when things aren't a good fit. I worked with a dentist, with a few years of an associateship under her belt with her search for a practice in the suburbs of Seattle. Married with a few kids, she and her husband spoke at length with me about the importance of good schools and a short commute. They wanted to raise their kids in an environment similar to their suburban upbringing. But, like a lot of doctors looking for a practice to buy, she was having trouble finding one that fit her criteria. She called me about a practice in downtown Seattle, outside her previous search range. We looked at the numbers of the practice, and the quantitative side of the analysis could work. However, I was concerned about her desire for a short commute given the practice location.

I asked her, "Where would you live if you bought this practice? Have you found a neighborhood close to the practice with good schools?"

(Long Pause)

"The closest one my husband and I feel comfortable with is 15 miles north of downtown." She replied sounding a little guarded.

Personally having been stuck in Seattle traffic many times, I responded, "That's…what?...a 30 minute drive on I-5 one way, on a good day, right?"

A second pause, "About that, yes."

"And about an hour in traffic, right?" was my follow up question.

Knowing what I was going to say next, she replied, "Or more."

I asked my last question, "So why are we even talking about this practice?"

Don't buy a practice, just because you're mentally ready to

move on to your next career step. Would you ever get married without dating first? Would you buy a car without at least taking it for a test drive? Would you buy a house without seeing and inspecting it first?

You've got to get out and see the practice first-hand. And when you do, there are seven areas to pay special attention to. I'll give you a few of the questions for each of the seven areas you need to ask when looking.

Key Area #1 – The Family Test

The Family Test could also be called the Monopoly Test because if the answer is "no" to any of the following questions, do not pass go and stop analyzing this practice. You're considering living somewhere for a period of, probably, decades. Consider the following questions:

- Can you live in this location, and (more importantly, if applicable) can your spouse live here?

- Will taxes and the cost of living here enhance or detract from your financial goals?

- Will you be able to do the things that are important to you if you spend 50 weeks a year in this part of the country?

Key Area #2 – The Selling Doctor

Interview the selling doctor; get to know him or her. If your style doesn't match the selling doctor, it will be more difficult to carry the practice forward in the way it has been carried so far. Consider these questions about the selling doctor:

- Do you and the seller have similar values?

- Is your personality style and approach with patients, staff and vendors similar to the selling doctor's?

- Are you comfortable with the seller's ethics?

- Is your clinical diagnosis philosophy similar to the seller's?

Key Area #3 – The Facility

Don't even think about purchasing a practice unless you have visited, or plan to visit the practice in person. There is no substitute for a boots-on-the-ground inspection of the facility, grounds, and area. Consider asking these questions as you consider the facility:

- What is your first impression of the physical appearance of the inside and outside of the building?

- Is the office and any signage easily visible?

- Would you be a dental patient in this office?

- Are there any major changes you'll need to make to the building soon after buying?

- Is there enough parking and will your patients be competing for parking spaces with other businesses?

Key Area #4 – The Equipment

The tools you'll be working with can enhance or detract from the practice you purchase. If you're a recent grad, you're probably familiar with the latest and greatest equipment most dental schools seem to have. Consider the following questions regarding equipment:

- Does the practice have all the instruments and equipment you'll need to do your work?

- If not, how much will it cost to purchase the equipment you need?

- Have you verified the equipment is left or right-handed?

- Is the behind the scenes equipment (compressor, vacuum, delivery units, nitrous, etc.) in good shape?

- Have you gotten the local equipment rep's opinion about the equipment?

Key Area #5 – The Team

Your team will be your family away from home. Getting along with them is important. But even more important is understanding who they are as individuals. Learn their reasons for being in their careers. Ask about their hopes, dreams and goals. Ask about their ability to be coached, and expectations of their new boss. Consider these questions as you analyze the team:

- Is the staff aware of the transition? How do they feel overall about the transition?

- Does the staff feel comfortable sharing their opinions of what is good about the practice and what they would change in the practice?

- What changes would they like to see in the practice? What are they anxious to keep unchanged?

- How long have members of the staff been with this office?

- Can you live with the current salaries, benefits and any existing employment contracts in place?

- How often do they receive feedback (both positive and negative)? How often do they improve their ability to contribute value to the practice?

- Do they know the practice goals? Do they have personal goals or development plans?

- Is everyone planning on staying after the transition? Who will you have to replace?

- What are the main reasons other staff have left this practice in the past?

Key Area #6 – The Patients & Scheduling

Patient flow and scheduling are the circulatory system of any practice. Without it, the practice dies. If there are problems with patients and scheduling, everything else becomes harder. Consider these questions when considering patients and scheduling:

- Is the doctor at least 70-80% booked for the next two weeks? How far out is the doctor fully booked?

- Is there room in the schedule for emergency visits?

- Does the hygiene schedule have any gaps? How far out is hygiene booked?

- What changes would you make to the scheduling process?

- Where do most new patients come from? How do they hear about the practice and decide to schedule an appointment?

- Are there any internal marketing programs? What do the seller and staff think about their effectiveness?

- Are there any external marketing programs? What do the seller and staff think about their effectiveness?

- What is your first impression of the practice's website? When was it last updated?

- What is the practice's online marketing plan? Does it include social media & SEO?

Key Area #7 – Production & Chart Audit

Patients may be coming in the doors, but how do you know they are the types of patients you will be able to help? Or the types of patients you want to help? Consider the following questions about the production and charts in the practice:

- What percentage of active patients pay via fee for service, PPO, HMO, and Medicaid?

- How much of total production comes from hygiene?

- Is the practice still using paper charts?

- Pull several charts and review the imaging and notes

and compare them with the work diagnosed and performed. Do you agree with how the patient was diagnosed and treated?

- Are the treatment notes legible and complete? Could you pick up this chart and treat the patient without trouble?

- Do you have the expertise to confidently perform the top 25 procedures by revenue and volume?

- How much accepted treatment is scheduled but not yet performed?

A final tip as you consider the list above: the help of a professional who specializes in helping dentists with this type of analysis is invaluable. Your dental accountant and attorney are your best resource. The bankers, brokers and equipment reps you're working with can help, too. Not only can they help you think through all of the above and more, they can give you a sense of what the answers to those questions mean. If the quantitative side of a practice analysis works, and the qualitative side in the questions above work, you may have found a practice worth buying!

> Need a second opinion of the qualitative factors of a practice you're considering buying? I am happy to help you. Schedule a free consultation at **www.BrianHanks.com/connect** because you understand the value of outsourcing to specialists.

Submitting an Offer and Letter of Intent

When buying a dental practice, one of the most important documents in the process is the Letter of Intent (or LOI, for short). The letter of intent is the legally non-binding document that contains all the elements of the practice transition you have negotiated with the seller. The letter of intent saves you money by allowing you to negotiate with the seller before you begin paying an attorney for drafting documents or other related services.

What is a Letter of Intent and What Does it Include?

The LOI is a written version of the key elements of the deal. It has the items that need to be negotiated with the seller in one place, written down and agreed to. Typically it is two to five pages long, depending on how much legalese is included. The document is typically signed by both the buyer and seller once you've agreed to the contents. It is expected portions of this document will be negotiated. If a broker gives you an LOI and tells you nothing is negotiable (or "it's not legally binding anyway, so what's the big deal?") than you are probably looking at a practice you should walk away from.

Typically an LOI is not legally binding, though some versions do contain a clause or two that legally binds the two parties to pursing the deal until the parties either finalize or walk away from the transaction. For example, the legally binding portion might include an exclusivity clause stating once you and the seller sign the LOI, the seller must take the practice off the market and not continue shopping it around while you work on due diligence, financing, etc.

Essentially, a letter of intent is a document that says, "The seller and I have talked, and we agreed to the following. We'd like the deal to look like this."

The LOI won't contain every important detail in the transaction—that's what the final legal purchase documents are for. They will contain the important stuff and anything with significant dollars on the line.

Why Getting the Letter of Intent Right is Crucial

Getting the Letter of Intent right typically leads to much smoother transactions where everyone is happy—the buyer, seller, staff, and patients. Getting the LOI right sets expectations for both parties up front.

I recently helped a buyer purchase a dental practice after the initial negotiations and Letter of Intent had been signed. I asked the buyer to send me a copy of the LOI. The price of the dental practice was on the paper, but not much else. Over the next few weeks, the buyer asked for deal elements that would ensure a smooth patient transition and help his tax situation. The seller was offended the buyer would "change the deal." The seller assumed because an LOI was signed, the buyer should just take whatever else was offered. The transition ended on a positive note, but with concessions the buyer didn't need to give, and not with some serious risk of the deal falling apart.

If the Letter of Intent is so important when buying a dental practice, how do you know what it should contain? How can you be sure you've negotiated the key elements and nothing is missing that might come back to bite you later on down the road?

What a Letter of Intent Should Include

Making sure the elements below are included is a key step in the process. A letter of intent for a dental transition should include *at a minimum* the following:

1. Included and excluded assets
2. Accounts Receivable and an A/R purchase schedule
3. Purchase price and tax asset allocation
4. Due diligence period
5. Intentions around real estate
6. Details around the seller's transition
7. What will happen with employees and benefits
8. Redos and rework
9. Restrictive covenants

Included and Excluded Assets

One dentist I talked with recently told me about the first day she showed up at the practice she purchased, only to find every single piece of furniture and fixture gone. Every couch. Every painting. The chairs the front desk had used for years—gone. Even the little potted plants around the office had walked away. She just assumed those were part of the transition. She spent the first few days making Costco and Ikea runs instead of being focused on the staff, patients, and processes in the office.

A good letter of intent will call out specifically which assets are included in the sale and which are not. Typically, included assets will be equipment, supplies, instruments, furniture, fixtures, computers, digital assets (website, phone number), etc.

Assets typically not included are cash, personal effects, employee benefits, liabilities of the seller, and any cars the practice might own.

Less important is the actual list. More important is that you and seller are on the same page and that you won't have any surprises.

Accounts Receivable and an A/R Purchase Schedule

You need to know if, and under what terms, you are purchasing accounts receivable. Not every seller wants to sell the accounts receivable, but many do. I recommend purchasing them if you can—if done correctly, it's like buying cash at a discount.

Most importantly, you need to spell out under what terms you'll purchase the accounts receivable. Typically, this looks like a table with the various aging categories and the value you will pay for them. You'll pay less for accounts receivable that have been outstanding longer because the risk is higher that you won't ever collect the money.

(Figure 2.7)

Example of Accounts Receivable Purchase Table

AR Age (days)	Rate:
0-30	85%
31-60	75%
61-90	50%
91-120	20%
120+	0%

If you don't purchase the accounts receivable, I recommend making it clear you are willing to collect and remit payment on the selling doctor's accounts. But you'll do it for a fee of around 5% of the value of those accounts collected. Collecting the selling doctor's money after the transition is fine, but it will take time, energy and resources away from *your* business and you should be compensated for going to the trouble.

Purchase Price and Tax Asset Allocation

Of course, you'll include the price of the practice in the Letter of Intent with the breakdown of the allocation of the total price. When purchasing a business, the IRS gives different tax treatment to the various assets being purchased—dental supplies, equipment, patient records, goodwill, etc. The next chapter has a more in-depth discussion on how to the asset allocation works and its tax implications.

The asset allocation is one of those negotiating areas where a win/win arrangement is tough. Typically, if the seller wins, the buyer loses and vice versa. There are a few areas where you can work out a mutually beneficial arrangement with the seller, but be aware of some of the tax basics in this section and be sure to use your dental accountant to help analyze what will work for you here.

As the buyer, you care about the asset allocation because how the purchase price is broken out will affect how quickly you can depreciate and write off the value of the practice you're buying. Thus, potentially lowering your tax bill.

As of 2016, the assets can be depreciated as follows in the table below. Lower numbers generally are better for you as the buyer (but not always, so talk with your accountant to know for sure).

(Figure 2.8)

Asset Type	Depreciation Period
Dental & Office Supplies	1 Year
Dental Equipment	7 Years
Leasehold Improvements	15 Years
Non-compete Covenant	15 Years
Patients Records	15 Years
Goodwill	15 Years

Due Diligence Period

Make sure you and the seller are clear on how long you and your dental accountant will need to review the practice and financial information. I typically recommend at least 30 days.

You'll also want to be specific about what access you and your dental accountant will need in order to complete the due diligence.

Intentions Around Real Estate

Are you going to buy the real estate? Are you going to rent from the seller? If renting, would you like the right of first refusal on the sale of the building? Don't leave those questions to chance and make sure they're spelled out in the Letter of Intent.

Details Around the Seller's Transition

Each situation will be unique, but you want to make sure the seller helps set you up for success as the buyer. You will want the seller to author a letter (that you help edit) informing patients from the last three or so years about the change in ownership and how amazing you as the buyer are. In fact, many state dental boards require this letter be written and sent. Spell out who is going to pay for the letter.

Also, you will want to talk with the seller about their availability post-transition to help understand the operations of the practice and possibly help with consultations in-person, or via telephone, email, etc.

Employees

One seller I know gave his employees all big raises between the time he agreed to sell the practice and the time the buyer took over. Staff compensation went from 28.5% of collections to 31.8%. I don't know for sure the motivation for the change, but you can be sure the buyer wasn't able to show up on the first day and say: "Just kidding everyone! Let's go back to your pay level from four months ago!"

Make clear to the seller all accrued benefits (bonuses, paid time off, etc.) are the responsibility of the seller before you take over the practice. I strongly, strongly recommend making as few changes to the staff, pay, benefits, etc. as possible in the first few months of business (with the one exception being the 401k or another pension plan). Make it clear to the seller you intend to keep all the staff, but all accrued benefits and promises are their responsibility.

Redos and Rework

Decide with the seller up front how you will handle patient cases that were originally handled by the seller but come back to your office to be fixed after you're the owner. Who will do the work? Who will pay for it?

If the seller hasn't left town, I like to see the seller have the option to come back in and do the work (of course, paying for staff time and materials required).

Restrictive Covenants

Make sure you negotiated upfront in the letter of intent the restrictive covenant the seller will be subject to. Include both the time and distance (e.g. 5 years and 15 miles) in the LOI. You will also want to include language around recruiting former employees and marketing within that same distance.

A good Letter of Intent is one of the keys to successfully buying a dental practice. You will minimize misunderstanding, maximize your use of time and energy, and possibly save money when you turn over a document to the lawyers that is complete and doesn't require a lot of back and forth.

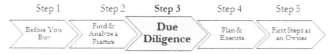

Step 1	Step 2	**Step 3**	Step 4	Step 5
Before You Buy	Find & Analyze a Practice	**Due Diligence**	Plan & Execute	First Steps as an Owner

- Financial Due Diligence
- Buyer Due Diligence
- Negotiations & Final Terms
- How to Get a Bank Loan

STEP 3:
DUE DILIGENCE

Knowing what you're getting is never more important than when buying a dental practice. This is one of the most expensive purchases you will ever make.

"Due Diligence" is a fancy accountant term for, "asking questions and checking data to make sure things are what someone else says they are." In the business world the term commonly refers to evaluating a business for sale.

One temptation at this stage will be to outsource the responsibility of due diligence to your team. You should have help, but, the ultimate responsibility is yours. Your dental accountant should perform a thorough review of all financial and tax records. The ultimate responsibility to understand exactly what you are buying is yours.

Use this guide during the site visit you schedule with the seller. Spend at least two days getting detailed answers to everything below so you can feel confident about your purchase.

Financial Due Diligence

Two parties will help you verify that the numbers reported to you from the seller or broker match what is actually happening in the practice. First, your dental accountant should look at the financial aspects of the practice using a checklist similar to the one below. The second party is the underwriting team of whichever bank you use to get your practice loan. You can read more about getting a bank loan later in this chapter on page XX.

Verify that your dental accountant reviews the financial aspects of the practice you're considering purchasing using the list below. Ask them their thoughts on these items. Get their opinion on insights gained about the practice after reviewing:

- **Tax Return Verification** – Do the amounts reported in a valuation or profit and loss statement match numbers reported to the IRS for the past four years?
- **Accounts Receivable** – How much is in the accounts receivable and how long has it been outstanding? What do the amounts say about operations of the business?
- **Production** – Which procedures drive the majority of production? Can the buyer perform them? Are there any procedures currently referred that the buyer can do?
- **Work Days** – How many total days were worked last year by the doctor? How many work days for the hygiene staff?
- **Lease** – Is the lease assignable? What are the financial commitments the buyer is taking on? Does the lease warrant a review by a lease specialist?
- **Employee Census** – How long have the employees worked at the practice and how typical is turnover?

What benefits and incentives are currently expected among staff?

- **Active Patients** – What is the seller's definition of active patients and how many do they have? How many received and accepted treatment plans?
- **Fee Analysis** – Where do the codes that produce the top 80% of revenue fall compared to others in the same zip code? When was the last time fees were raised?

Again, your dental accountant should help provide you answers to all the questions above. Much of the information will be provided by the seller or broker (if available). You may need to request reports from the seller or seller's team.

Buyer Due Diligence

After you've signed the Letter of Intent but before you've signed closing documents is the time to kick the tires, take the test drive, and make sure you know exactly what you're buying.

A physical on-site visit of a dental practice is non-negotiable before you buy the practice. If you already work in the practice, you're already familiar with what happens on a day-to-day basis in the practice. Everyone else needs to plan to spend at least two days on-site reviewing the practice.

Sometimes a broker or seller will push back against a site visit, or try to time a site visit for a time when the staff isn't around. The desire in these situations is to keep the sale of the practice quiet to avoid any negative repercussions from staff who could leave or patients who may leave.

Push back hard against the requirement to only visit the practice outside of business hours. Assuming that you've signed an LOI, are securing financing, and have engaged an accountant and attorney, you've shown adequate commitment to the purchase. You deserve the opportunity to see the practice in action, watch patient/staff interactions, see the processes and procedures of the business you'll be running, and get to know the people you'll be working with.

Every situation is unique, so lean on your advisors for specific advice if you get pushback on visiting when the practice is open.

The end goal of your buyer due diligence visit is to answer every question listed in the seven sections of "How to Analyze the Qualitative Factors" in Chapter 2.

Negotiating Tips For Buying a Dental Practice

I recently experienced a parenting moment that reminded me of negotiations when buying a dental practice, and how quickly things can go badly.

I had promised each of the kids a small bag of M&Ms after work. I followed through and delivered. I tallied the dad points in my head. I then watched as the 2-year-old ripped open the bag and one of the green M&Ms escaped and fell, rolling onto the floor. Of course.

The 3-year-old was fast.

She jumped down, snagged it, and popped it in her mouth in full view of the 2-year-old who still had an entire bag of chocolate happiness, minus one escapee.

I'm sure you can guess what happened next.

The 2-year-old dissolved in tears and decided to throw a fit. One lost M&M made her so angry the rest of the bag in front of her didn't even register.

This is the very definition of a scarcity mindset. If you've read Steven Covey's *7 Habits of Highly Effective People* you remember this principle. Dr. Covey outlines how zero sum thinking makes people sad, jealous, and greedy. Scarcity makes you think there are only so many M&Ms in the world, and if you share any of them with *anyone* you'll miss out and starve to death. This kind of thinking happens when negotiating buying a dental practice all the time.

It's the kind of thinking that can ruin a perfectly good deal.

Most often when negotiating buying a dental practice it happens around the purchase price. The selling doctor gets a price in their head of what their practice is worth, and throws a fit when they receive an offer that is less than what they think they "deserve." I know of one selling dentist who almost derailed a deal over $5,000 on a purchase price of over $1.5 Million. A single M&M rolling away is the perfect analogy for a deal like that.

But what if you are buying a dental practice, and you don't think the practice is worth what the selling doctor wants? What if you love the practice, would love to buy, but you've talked with the seller or broker and have been told "there is absolutely no wiggle room on price!" (Let's assume, for this example, that's actually true.) And, then, your dental accountant is telling you the practice is <u>not</u> worth what the seller wants. What now?

Answer: find other deal points to negotiate where real dollars are at stake and might soften the blow to you of overpaying.

Let's look at an example.

Let's say you're looking at a great dental practice for sale in the city where you want to live, with a phenomenal staff, great patient base and an office location that is *perfect*. The seller wants $1,000,000 for the practice and won't take a penny less. Your dental accountant is telling you the practice is only worth $900,000.

$100,000 is a big difference. What now?

If you were to say, "Oh well. I guess this is what I have to pay…" your monthly payments on a 10-year, 4% loan would increase from $9,112 to $10,125 – over $1,000 a month in cash flow you could use to invest in the practice, or use at home to pay down student loans.

Not only would you pay $100,000 more in the *principal* on the loan, but your total *interest* payments over the life of the loan would increase from $193,447 to $214,942 – an additional $21,494 you're paying the bank on the larger amount the seller wants.

Are you stuck? Are you out of options? Do you suck it up and overpay?

Luckily, no.

Step into my dental accounting office, let me get out my green eyeshade and calculator, and allow me to introduce you to two topics where you can get some of the difference back.

The two additional areas where you can negotiate buying a dental practice that will put real dollars in your pocket, besides the asking price are (1) buying the accounts receivable, and (2) the asset allocation. I'll talk about the former in this section, and the latter in the next.

Negotiation Opportunity: Accounts Receivable

When you purchase a practice, you are buying an income stream. The day you own the practice, there will still be patients that owe the practice money. The seller owns the money that is still owed. But you can buy that money owed the seller by offering to purchase the accounts receivable (A/R).

When you pull an accounts receivable report from the practice management software system, the system will separate the total accounts receivable into different "vintages." Current accounts receivable is for any procedure done in the last 30 days, the next oldest is for anything 31-60 days old, and so on.

It can be a hassle for the seller to keep track of and ultimately collect on the accounts receivable, so often the buyer will offer to purchase the accounts receivable, usually at a discount.

In the Letter of Intent, the buyer will offer to purchase the accounts receivable on a sliding scale that reflects the format of the system generated A/R aging report. The scale will reflect the fact that "fresher" bills are more likely to be paid, and bills that have been outstanding for a while may never be paid.

Buying the accounts receivable is like offering to buy a

stack of money for a slightly shorter stack of money.

And the seller is usually happy to make the trade because you're relieving her of the *responsibility* of collecting the money—she can make a clean break from the practice after the sale! Additionally, banks typically will add on to the practice loan the amount needed to purchase the A/R.

Back to our example.

Let's assume the $1,000,000 practice has $100,000 in outstanding accounts receivable, broken out into the buckets or "vintages" in the table below.

(Figure 3.1)

Accounts Receivable Example

AR Age (days)	Amount
0-30	$75,000
31-60	$15,000
61-90	$7,500
91-120	$1,500
120+	$1,000
	$100,000

So, the buyer would offer a percentage discount off the amounts in those buckets of accounts receivable. Typically, in a letter of intent, the A/R offer will take the form of a table similar to this one.

(Figure 3.2)
Accounts Receivable Example with Offer Applied

AR Age (days)	Amount	Rate:	Offer
0-30	$75,000	85%	$63,750
31-60	$15,000	75%	$11,250
61-90	$7,500	50%	$3,750
91-120	$1,500	20%	$300
120+	$1,000	0%	$0
	$100,000		$79,050

Applying those percentages to our example of $100,000 in accounts receivable yields the result of ultimately paying $79,050 for $100,000. Remember we felt like we were overpaying for this practice by $100,000. By offering to buy the accounts receivable, we've made up $21,000 of the difference already!

Of course, every purchase will have its own specific numbers. The amount of accounts receivable on the books of a practice will vary greatly from practice to practice. Ironically for our example, having a *low* amount of accounts receivable is a good thing – a sign of a healthy practice collecting quickly on the dental work it performs! (Which, incidentally, *could* be one reason why the seller feels justified in a higher asking price!)

The point here isn't the math. The point is that when you feel stuck with an asking price higher than you feel like you want to pay as a buyer, *one way* to feel better about the deal and to feel like you are coming away with some real dollars in the negotiations is to offer the seller to make a clean break from the practice, and negotiate favorable terms to buy the accounts receivable.

Negotiation Opportunity: Asset Allocation

Another area where significant dollars can change hands when buying a dental practice is the asset allocation, or tax treatment, of the total purchase price. You don't need to become a tax expert, but a little knowledge here can go a long way toward coming together with a seller on a deal.

Asset allocation is an accounting term. Asset allocation is a fancy way to say how much value the accountants in the deal are assigning to the different items being purchased.

"But I'm only buying one thing," you may say, "a dental practice!"

Not true, says the Internal Revenue Service (IRS).

When you buy a pair of shoes in the store you really are only buying one "thing." It's a one-for-one exchange. Money for a sweet pair of kicks.

When you buy a business, however, you're paying for multiple different *types* of assets. You're buying supplies, equipment, goodwill, and so on.

(Figure 3.3)

Typical Asset Allocation for a Dental Practice Transition

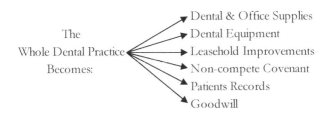

The primary reason the asset allocation matters on your (the buyer's) side is that the IRS allows different depreciation time periods for different asset types. Depreciation is easy to understand with a quick example. Pretend you stumbled upon a genie right after graduating dental school. One of the wishes the genie offered you is for your first job as a dentist to pay you for the next five years of work *all in advance*.

(Ignore for a minute your stunningly inept ability to think of *better* wishes and go with this example.)

There you are, the morning of your first day as a real dentist, gigantic check in hand and feeling good. You've got a pile of money and haven't had to work for it yet. Honest person you are, you are still going to show up to work and work just as hard as if the owner was just paying you as you go.

But what about the owner? Does she get to say she had a gigantic expense in year one and avoid taxes that year?

Nope.

The IRS would apply depreciation rules to my completely ridiculous example and only allow the owner to count 1/5 of that gigantic check of yours for each of the next five years. After all, the gigantic paid-in-advance check is for your next five year's work.

The same principle applies to any asset you purchase as a business owner that has a value of more than $600 and a useful life of more than a year. For example, when you buy a computer, you're probably going to use it for more than 1 year, and as such there are rules about how much of the computer's price you get to expense on each year's tax return.

Depreciation is the rule that allocates value to a tangible asset over its useful life. It's an attempt by the IRS to match the *expense* of an item to the *revenue* the asset helps you earn.

Typically, the depreciation rules break the assets of a dental practice into the three main buckets seen in the images below.

(Figure 3.4)

Asset Allocation Depreciation for Buyer

Asset Category	Depreciation Period
Dental & Office Supplies	1 Year
Dental Equipment	5-7 Years
Leasehold Improvements	15 Years
Non-compete Covenant	15 Years
Patients Records	15 Years
Goodwill	15 Years

How does this affect the seller? The seller doesn't care about depreciation, so why not try and just load everything into the categories most helpful to you as the buyer? Let's stick everything in Dental and Office Supplies and Dental Equipment!

Not so fast.

On the other side of the transaction, the IRS has different rules for the seller for the tax treatment of different assets sold.

The IRS has two ways to tax sales of assets where the seller makes money: ordinary income and long-term capital gains. Let's look at *ordinary income* first. This is the type of tax most people are familiar with. The ordinary income tax rates start at 10% and go up to a whopping 39.6%!

The second way the IRS taxes gains on asset sales is called *capital gains*. The basic theory behind capital gains is the IRS wants to reward people who invested in resources productive for society, like a business, with a lower overall tax rate on any gains from those investments.

The difference between the two is substantial, anywhere from 0% for low-income taxpayers to 20% for those in the top tax bracket.

(Figure 3.5)
Asset Allocation Tax Treatment for Seller

Asset Category	Depreciation Period
Dental & Office Supplies	Ordinary Income
Dental Equipment	Ordinary Income
Leasehold Improvements	Long-Term Capital Gain
Non-compete Covenant	Ordinary Income
Patients Records	Long-Term Capital Gain
Goodwill	Long-Term Capital Gain

If you are a seller, the obvious takeaway from this difference is that you want as much of your income to fall in an asset category where the IRS will tax it as *capital gains*, and not *ordinary income*. Doing this could save you as much as 20% on whatever money you can move from an ordinary income category to a capital gains category. The potential savings if you are the buyer are huge!

(Figure 3.6)

Capital Gains vs Ordinary Income - 2018 Federal Income Brackets

Individuals	Married Filing Jointly	Federal Income Tax Rate	Long-term Capital Gains Rate*
$9,525	$19,050	10%	0%
$38,700	$77,400	12%	0%
$82,500	$165,000	22%	15%
$157,500	$315,000	32%	15%
$200,000	$400,000	35%	15%-20%
$500,000	$600,000	37%	20%

* Plus 3.8% marginal medicare surtax if total income above applicable threshold

An important point to consider is that the buyer and seller are required to be consistent in how they treat the values in the different categories. You and the seller are both required to report these numbers to the IRS independently on your next year's tax return. While the numbers must match, the actual amounts allocated to the different assets is negotiable.

What are the rules? What does the law say? Per the IRS, the technical way to allocate the purchase price among the different assets is to allocate the Fair Market Value to the identifiable assets (patient records, equipment, supplies, etc.), then the remainder, if any, is allocated to Goodwill.

Many buyers assume the values assigned to the different categories are predetermined and set in stone. However, the definition of "Fair Market Value" is the price an independent buyer and seller can agree upon. So basically, if you and the seller agree on the price allocated to the assets, that price is correct.

Back to the point. As the buyer, you're looking for opportunities to negotiate with the seller on more than just the asking price. Ideally, there are lots of different areas where your interests overlap, or at least aren't directly opposed to one another. We now have three categories with significant dollars behind them where the buyer and seller can move levers to find the option that works best for everyone and leaves everyone happy: price, accounts receivable, and asset allocation.

For example, Dr. Seller could feel very strongly she wants a full-price offer on the practice she's worked hard to build over the last 25 years. Dr. Seller is going to be on the golf course a lot with her dentist friends and wants to be able to say she got a full price offer for her practice.

Dr. Buyer could ask if she would be willing come down in the percentage of the sale in the goodwill category and increase the amount allocated to equipment to allow her to depreciate the total cost of the sale more quickly.

Alternatively, Dr. Seller might be very sensitive about the large tax bill coming when he sells his practice. "No problem," says Dr. Buyer, "if you can come down in price a bit, I would be willing to increase the asset allocation of goodwill to allow you to have more of the sale taxed as long-term capital gains."

I've seen this happen frequently. Everyone walks away feeling like their needs are addressed and ultimately more satisfied with the deal.

Other Things to Negotiate When Buying a Dental Practice

Purchase price, accounts receivable and asset allocation are not the only items you can negotiate when buying a dental practice. They're the main items with real dollars behind them. But what if you need a little more ammunition as the buyer? What if you need a little extra push to get a seller on board with a plan that works well for you?

Other common areas of negotiation include:

- Start date
- Letter to active patients
- How to handle current employees
- Right of first refusal on the purchase of the building
- Redos
- Restrictive Covenant
- Deposit

If there's one eternal truth I've seen when helping buyers purchase a dental practice, it's this: The more knowledge and more options there are, the higher the chance of pulling together a deal.

Ultimately, most buyers and sellers want the same thing. They want to successfully transition the business into new, responsible hands that will take great care of the staff and patients. They want to be rewarded for all the hard work they've done to that point – the seller with a gigantic check and the buyer with a steady income stream from a healthy business.

You're more likely to get a win/win with a seller if you know what you can negotiate. Price is always negotiable. Purchasing the accounts receivable is a good negotiating point too. A great third option with real dollars behind it is the asset allocation. Know a few of the basics and work with your dental accountant to advise you on how you can profitably negotiate with the seller and create a situation where everyone wins.

How to Get a Loan

Buying a practice is, hopefully, something you'll do just once in your lifetime and you'll probably need to know how to get a dental practice loan to make it happen. Some dentists fear that with how much they owe in student loans they'll never qualify for a practice loan.

The truth of the matter is, if you're a dentist with at least one year of experience, a decent credit score, and a demonstrated ability to produce some dentistry, chances are good you won't have a problem getting a loan.

But how do you make sure you're getting the right loan? And how do you know you're getting the best deal?

Your Lending Options and How Banks See You

Here's the first thing to know about borrowing money to buy a dental practice: Banks think of dentists as a low risk loan. In fact, according to several bankers I've talked with dentists are *very* low risk. Dentistry is profitable and dentists nearly always pay back their loans.

For this reason, if you look at buying a healthy dental practice and you have a decent credit history, you shouldn't have a problem getting a good loan. Whether or not you get the loan will all come down to cash flow. Does the revenue that the practice collects after paying expenses cover not just your personal debts but leave enough to live on?

There are no guarantees, of course, but generally the hardest part about the lending process is choosing which loan proposal to accept.

There are several banks that have dental-specific lending

arms. These groups understand the unique economics of dental practices and lend accordingly. If you use one of these banks, you won't have trouble finding someone to work with.

Using a dental-specific lender has several key advantages.

1. **Specialty** - There are lenders who ONLY specialize in dental lending. Period. Those lenders know how a practice should run, and are your advocate if the deal works or doesn't work. Lenders who don't specialize in dental lending position the loan as a commercial loan. This can lead to hiccups as the cash flow and operations of a dental practice can look very different from other types of businesses.

2. **Speed** - You'll likely get a loan faster than working with a non-dental-specific lender.

3. **Amount** - Dental-specific lenders typically loan a larger amount of the purchase price than traditional small business lenders. Currently, most dental lenders will lend 100% of the purchase price and will often lend more for working capital or purchasing the accounts receivable. This is typically based on the revenues compared to the purchase price. Lenders tend to go up to 85% of last year's collections. Anything over that and the practice is considered to be selling at a premium. More on this number below.

4. **Advice** - Good dental lenders will know good practices from bad. They will help you think through the pros and cons of your practice. They can provide perspective and connect you to other service providers who specialize in your type of transaction.

How Banks Typically Make You an Offer

When you're choosing a lender it's important to understand a few of the basics of how dental lenders are structured and how their process works. Typically, there is a separation between the sales and underwriting teams. The sales folks are usually the ones you're talking with and the underwriters are often the ones who make a final decision on whether to lend you money.

That's not to say the sales folks don't know anything and aren't helpful. The opposite has been the case in my experience. The lenders who work on the sales side tend to be very helpful, quick to respond, and excellent at picking out what elements of a deal will be troublesome or problematic. Put your best foot forward when dealing with everyone at a bank.

Usually the process to get a practice loan will include three main steps:

1. **Application and document submission -** Each bank will have a different application that will ask basic questions about the amount you are applying to borrow, your background, the practice, and your plans as the owner. A key step in this process will be getting tax returns and financial documents to the bank. Your broker, dental accountant, or even the seller can help with this step if needed.

2. **Underwriting -** This is where the bank's team of analysts will look at the key financial data of both the practice and you as the borrower. They put it all in their gigantic computer and see what pops out. In a very real sense, the bank's underwriting team is performing your financial due diligence. Each lender has a different risk tolerance when it comes to underwriting. Some will do just a basic revenue/expense calculation. Others are more

detailed in their analysis, and can give you feedback on the depth of the analysis. An important point to remember is that if one bank declines the loan and one approves the loan, more than likely the bank who declined the loan did a deeper analysis due to their specialty. Be very cautious about accepting a loan from one bank when another declines to lend.

3. **Phone interview -** Usually the bank will have a member of the underwriting team get on the phone with you to talk about your background, history in dentistry, and goals as the practice owner. They'll be looking for information on how you handle money, how much experience you are bringing to the table, and your ideas for business ownership. Again, put your best foot forward and be honest.

Be aware there are the two types of loan proposals banks give you. Even if you have a loan proposal from a bank in hand, you must know what type it is.

Approach 1: Quick & Unapproved

Some banks will get a written proposal on the table as quickly as possible. In this scenario, your deal has *not* gone through underwriting yet and the terms are *close* to what underwriting will approve, but not finalized. The key advantage to this approach is speed and your ability to show a seller than you can get financing. Obviously, the downside to this approach is that the terms on the page could change after the underwriting team looks at the deal.

Some lenders will provide you with verbal confirmation of a loan amount over the phone. This is not an approval. It is a sales pitch to get you in the door. A lender giving you a verbal pre-approval for $500K is not providing a blank check to then use to shop for a practice. (This is yet another area where buying a dental practice is very different from buying a home.) It's entirely possible to receive approval for one practice at $750K, but get declined for a practice that is only $350K. Each approval is specific to the cash flow and economics of that one practice.

Approach 2: Slower & Approved

Other banks will get your info through underwriting, and make the first written offer the approved one. The main disadvantage to this approach is how long it takes to get you a written proposal to show the seller and make a plan for timing and expectations. But, you have final terms written down on paper, approved, and locked in. If you choose the lender that takes this approach, typically the deal can move very quickly after you commit.

It's important to remember that "slower" is not a synonym for "worse." Remember different banks have different underwriting standards. One bank can provide a quick approval, and another bank can ask for more information. A request for more information typically means the underwriter found some items that could be potential issues. They are red-flagging items that could burn you as the future owner. As infuriating as repeated questions can feel, usually it's in your best interest to remember that the reason for the extra time is to protect your investment.

What Banks Look at When Deciding Whether to Lend

The bank has one real concern: are they going to get paid back?

So how do they decide that?

Each of the different bankers I've worked with share similar numbers to describe what specifically their underwriting teams look at when considering a dental lending deal: 60% of the decision to give you a loan has to do with the practice, and 40% of the decision has to do with you personally as the borrower.

60% of the Decision – the Practice Numbers

On the practice side of the deal, the bank will look at the numbers below and feed them into the cash flow model. They'll use this model to project how much money you'll make as an owner of the practice you're considering, and if you can afford to make the required loan payments.

- **Collections** – How big is the practice? Are collections growing or shrinking?
- **Profitability** – How much of each dollar of collections does the doctor keep after paying all the expenses of the business?
- **Hygiene Production** – What percentage of total production comes from hygiene? What percentage comes from new patients? Returning patients?
- **Procedure Mix** – Can the purchasing doctor perform the same procedures the selling doctor performs? How much is being referred out?

Generally speaking, dental lenders will lend 100% of the purchase price of the practice plus an additional amount for either working capital or money to purchase the accounts receivable. This is true at nearly every bank I've worked with one crucial caveat: the 85% rule.

Banks will rarely lend a total of 85% of the prior year collections to buy a practice.

Put another way, if a practice collected exactly $1,000,000

last year, and you're buying the practice, the maximum amount that banks will lend you is $850,000 for the purchase price AND anything additional, like working capital and money to purchase the accounts receivable or to purchase new equipment.

The 85% number is definitely a rule of thumb, and generally the top limit. Practices *should* (always a dangerous word) sell for much less than that, on average. If you're borrowing 85% of the previous year's collections, you're probably buying a premium, top-of-the-line practice.

40% of the Decision – Your Creditworthiness

Now, over to the personal side. What specifically about YOU will the banks look at?

While the majority of the decision to lend you money will depend on the economics of the practice, you still have to have solid credit to get a loan for hundreds of thousands of dollars. Your dental degree is not reason enough.

First, the bank will run your credit. Make sure your credit score is 700 or above.

Second, the bank will look to see if you're responsible with money. Their best proxy for that metric is to ask how much cash you currently have. A good rule of thumb of cash to have on hand is 8-10% of the purchase price of the practice you're considering. If you don't know the size of the practice you'll eventually buy, shoot for somewhere between $25,000 and $50,000 of cash on hand. The bank probably won't make you put that money into the deal (if you're under the 85% threshold). They're looking for a sense of whether you spend every cent that hits your account or not. This money is also a safety net in case during your first week of ownership your payroll, supplies, the electricity, and rent bills come due at the same time a pipe bursts. No business owner should buy a business without having a safety net.

Third, the bank will look at your production history. They will want to know if you have the hand speed and clinical skills to perform the dentistry you will be doing in the practice you're going to buy. You do need to show that you have *already* produced close to the amount of production of the practice you're considering buying. But, the numbers will need to be close enough to tell a story as to why you'll be able to get close to what the seller is doing. Get and keep track of your production reports for the last six to twelve months. If you don't have them, ask your employer to provide them for your records. If you don't know your own production numbers how are you going to know what size of practice you can handle as an owner?

What if you have a blemish on your credit history somewhere in the past, like a short sale on a home or something similar? What if you've been aggressively paying down student loans and don't have much cash on hand? Never fear. Those rules of thumbs aren't deal breakers. They will be black marks that you'll need to have a good explanation for. If you know the question is coming, you can prepare accordingly and explain your unique situation.

How To Negotiate The Best Deal For Yourself with the Bank

In any negotiation, the person with the most options usually comes away with the better deal. The same is true when getting a bank loan to buy a practice.

If you can get approved from one bank, chances are good at least one more will give you a loan proposal. To get the best deal possible, get at least two offers from two different banks. Get written loan proposals from both. Then, ask your dental accountant to run the numbers and compare the two options. No two proposals will be the same. Each lender has a different reputation , parameters, fees, and terms. You need to consider all factors, including whether that lender will work with your advisors to provide a smooth ride to the finish line.

I've never seen a bank lead with their very best offer with the first loan proposal. But, I've also never seen a bank offer a better rate without another bank's offer on the table. I suggest talking with at least two banks but no more than four. Any incremental benefit you'd see from talking with five or more banks gets negated by the fact that whichever bank you're talking with knows the likelihood of you choosing them gets lower and lower the more banks you entertain.

Don't make the mistake of assuming banks will never know you're talking to their competitors. Those credit inquiries are visible on your credit report. Plus, most of the bankers know each other and they run into each other enough to compare notes about which buyers to avoid. You'll need bankers throughout your career. Don't burn bridges.

When you do get the loan, be on the lookout for more than just the interest rate. Make sure you look at the term (how many years you have to pay back the loan), the prepayment penalty requirements, and any fees. Also, don't forget to watch for any ancillary requirements like a mandatory requirement to use that bank's business checking account, for example.

I highly recommend using an experienced dental accountant through the negotiation process. If you work with someone with a track record, they'll know what the bankers want to see, where they could perhaps give a little, and what differences between loan terms really matter.

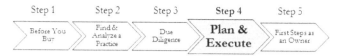

Step 1	Step 2	Step 3	Step 4	Step 5
Before You Buy	Find & Analyze a Practice	Due Diligence	**Plan & Execute**	First Steps as an Owner

• Pre-Ownership Checklist
• Avoid Common Mistakes

STEP 4:
EXECUTE THE TRANSITION AND PLAN FOR OWNERSHIP

You've signed an LOI and passed the stressful negotiations stage of buying a practice. You've completed the buyer due diligence and your dental accountant has completed the financial due diligence. Soon you'll be walking through the front doors of a practice you own. Congrats!

There is a lot to do between finalizing negotiations, lending and legal documents. But how do you know if you've completed all the details needed before you step in and run the business? How do you maximize the chances that the first few weeks in your new business will be positive?

What if you show up on your first day, like a pediatric dentist I know in Arizona, and you realize the schedule is only half-full, and your front desk can't bill to insurance yet because credentialing hasn't happened?

What if you're like an orthodontist in Texas who had to keep pushing back the close date on his practice three times because the bank wouldn't release funds due to lack of life and disability insurance?

What if you're like a general dentist I know in Seattle who showed up on his first day of ownership to find out two of his five employees had quit, and weren't coming back?

With a little knowledge of what is left to do, you can feel confident. You can feel ready. You can walk through those doors on day one knowing you've taken care of the essentials and you're ready to wow your patients and continue an amazing career.

Everything Else to Do Before Closing

Step 1: Make Sure Your Dental License is in Place

While obvious, some buyers I've talked with don't know that the bank won't lend you the money you need to buy your practice if your state license is not in place. This can take a while (Florida is the worst, from what I've seen) so get started on you state license right away!

Step 2: Finalize Your Financing

Work closely with your accountant to help you find the best lenders, apply to them, and evaluate the offers they provide. I recommend buyers evaluate at least two different lending offers. Have your dental accountant evaluate the offers, because the best option may not be the one with the lowest interest rate! There is a whole chapter with details on this step, in case you're skipping around. Read more on how to get a bank loan in Chapter 3.

Step 3: Start on Your Life and Disability Insurance Policies

Like your state dental license, getting life and disability policies in place can take a while. Evaluate multiple quotes, and use your accountant to help you decide which options are best for you and your situation. And which will fit your budget. The bank you choose will have you "collaterally assign" the benefits of these policies to them. This means the bank will get paid before you or your spouse do. Don't make the mistake of assuming just because they bank says you have enough insurance you're properly covered. Work with your dental accountant to make sure you understand what would happen should the unthinkable take place and to be properly insured.

Step 4: Plan Your Buyer Due Diligence Trip

Visiting the practice, and working with the seller *before* signing the letter of intent is a lot like dating – everyone has their best foot forward. You must take a separate due diligence trip to the practice after signing the letter of intent. You will visit to evaluate, in depth, items like: equipment, building, signage, patient charts, scheduling, employees, accounts receivable, etc.

I send my buyers with a 5-page document chock full of questions about the practice the buyer should know. The questions cover everything from patient charts, equipment, the building, signage, the staff and more. This usually takes buyers two days to complete. We then review the document to ensure that what the buyer saw, is what they expected. We ensure there will be no surprises when they show up as the owner.

Step 5: Get Your Contents, Malpractice & Business Insurance Policies in Place

Work with an insurance agent to make sure your business insurance policies are in place, as well as your life and disability. Business insurances don't typically take as long as life and disability to nail down, but are still crucial.

Step 6: Get Credentialed with All the Seller's Accepted Insurance Plans

You'll want to be able to bill, and collect as soon as possible. One key to making that happen is to be credentialed with all the insurance providers the seller's patients currently use. Be ready for lots of phone calls and emails here, but this is important and should not be put off! Business survival is all about cash flow, and cash will come into the business when you can bill your patients' insurance providers and get checks mailed to you!

Step 7: Set Up Your Business Entity

Work with your accountant and attorney to determine which type of business entity is best for your situation. You have two options to file with your state for your business entity:

Option 1: Do it yourself with a service like legalzoom.com. The advantage here is it's generally a little cheaper to do this on your own. Unless you feel confident you know what you're doing, there can be a steep learning curve that probably isn't worth climbing for most dentists.

Option 2: Utilize your attorney. Any good dental attorney will have included entity set up as part of their package. If you've chosen an attorney with a flat rate, this won't cost you anything additional. Logistically, this step is not very difficult. It's definitely worth outsourcing this task to someone else who has done it hundreds of times and recommend letting a lawyer tackle this step.

Step 8: Establish Your Business Banking Accounts

Get your business bank accounts set up quickly after your letter of intent is signed. You'll want to be ready to collect money, pay bills, payroll and other expenses and need to have an account to pay those from. Second, keep track of any and all business-related expenses between now and ownership. After negotiations, but before taking ownership is the perfect time to separate business and personal expenses. Your accountant can go back and re-categorize the two if they are mixed, but keeping things separate early on will make your life easier.

One suggestion with your business checking account: if you don't have any objection, go with the biggest bank in your area. Typically, this will be Wells Fargo, Chase or Bank of America. Their business checking solutions are generally very good, and they have lots of physical locations if you need to visit a branch. Finally, their online access for accountants is almost always far superior to the local credit union or small bank on the corner. Superior technology makes delegation of your finances to other parties much, much simpler.

Step 9: Have Your Accountant File Business Info with IRS

You'll typically need to file two forms with the IRS when starting your dental practice business. First, your new dental practice will need an Employer Identification Number (EIN). This is like your personal social security number, but for your business. You'll use this number a lot. This is IRS Form SS-4 and your accountant can fill it out for you and get your signature before submitting. Second, as long as your accountant and lawyer agree and help you select an LLC taxed as an S-corporation, your business will need to file IRS form 2553. This elects "selection" taxation for your LLC. Ask your accountant for details, but you essentially get the legal liability protection of an LLC, with the taxation benefits of an s-corporation.

Step 10: Work With a Payroll Company to Ensure State IDs Are In Place

Before you show up to the office on day one, you need to ensure you have a plan to pay your employees. As an employer, nearly every state will require you have what's called a "state employer ID." Your payroll company can help here.

Make life simple on yourself. Hire a payroll company to take care of getting your employees paid. Your payroll company will help you decide on payroll frequency. They'll provide the software. They'll help file quarterly state payments, and will handle any notifications you get from the state or federal government. Your payroll company will also ensure you've filed all the necessary paperwork to have the right identification numbers on file with the state and federal government.

Step 11: Sign Lease & Asset Purchase Agreements

Your attorney will help you with the review and collaboration on the documents that will officially transfer ownership of the dental practice to you and your business entity. Yes, this is one of those times in life you need to read every word of those long documents. Sorry! Muscle through, and use a highlighter. Ask your accountant or attorney questions about sections and language you don't understand. Be crystal clear about what you're agreeing to!

Step 12: Ensure Accountant Verifies Form 8594 With Seller's Accountant

When you buy a business, typically the sales price will be broken up into different types of assets – supplies, equipment, goodwill, etc. This is called the "asset allocation". When you file your next tax return, your accountant will include that information with your return. The IRS will compare the information you include with the seller's tax return and ensure the two asset allocation amounts line up. The name of this form is Form 8594. Make sure your accountant coordinates with the seller's accountant to ensure the two line up.

Step 13: Set Up Merchant Services Account

Merchant services is a fancy way to say you have a credit card reader in your office, and can take credit and debit card payments from patients. Obviously, the ability to accept payments from patients is why you're in business. There are a couple dental-specific merchant services providers that do a fantastic job for dentists. Ask your accountant which one they recommend. Getting set up is typically quick, and can be done is less than a week.

Step 14: Meet With the Staff, Change Nothing

Set up a meeting with the staff of your new practice and get to know them. For many dentists, you'll spend more time with your staff than you will with your family. Start to build those great relationships! Meet one on one with these folks and ask about what is important to them. What do they live for? What do they like about the office? What they would change about the office?

You'll have lots of ideas on how to improve the way the dental practice runs. Staff-related improvements should be on the list, <u>but delayed</u>! Don't make changes to staff, salary, benefits, vacation, etc. for at least the first 90 days of owning your practice. (The exception to this rule is a pension or 401k plan. It's important to start your own, and not adopt the previous owner's plan. Talk to your dental accountant for details.)

Your staff knows the patients. Your staff knows the processes of the practice. Helping them to feel comfortable with the change in doctor will go a long way towards ensuring patient turnover stays low and your first few months of business lay the solid foundation for even better results down the road.

You can read more details on this topic in chapter 5.

Step 15: Celebrate!

Finally, take an evening or two to celebrate with your significant other or close friends. Buying a dental practice is a big deal! You've worked your tail off to get into and finish dental school. Odds are, you have worked hard as an employee or associate somewhere before owning your practice. You've had a long road to get to where you are! You're probably not diving into piles of money Scrooge-McDuck-style yet, but you absolutely should spend a little and celebrate the amazing accomplishment of getting to where you are today!

Walking through the doors of a dental practice you own *should* be a feeling of accomplishment and excitement! The last thing you want to feel on that day is a sense of dread or worry over some detail you haven't yet completed. Make sure your team has helped you through a checklist similar to the one above to ensure you're ready to start strong in your new practice!

How to Avoid Common Mistakes Buying a Practice

I've worked with a lot of clients to help them successfully transition to dental practice ownership. I'm proud of my track record with my clients, and the results of the good work I've done to ensure both the buyer and seller are happy with the transition. I've seen, from time to time, a few common dental practice transition mistakes.

As I lay out the most common mistakes, I've added a simple question or two you can ask a potential seller as you shop different practice. By the way, if a seller or broker acts offended or put out you would ask any of these questions, feel free to throw me under the bus. "Sorry. I read a book by this guy who said I needed to ask these questions." These are questions too important *not* to ask.

Mistake #1 - Seller Not Actually Ready to Sell

This first type comes up more frequently than you'd imagine. In a nutshell, some sellers are mentally ready to sell before they are financially able. A seller in Washington State wanted to sell his practice, but had not reviewed his finances to see if he could afford to walk away from dentistry yet. The seller retained a broker, listed the practice, and my client became interested and engaged me. I helped the buyer perform due diligence on the practice, and the buyer flew out to the practice to look things over. The buyer put together an offer with my help and submitted it to the seller's broker. After the broker and seller received the offer, the seller talked with his accountant and learned even if he sold at that price, he would need to be on a rice and beans diet for the rest of his life if he wanted to retire right then.

The seller backed out to the considerable annoyance (and wasted time and money) of everyone else involved.

Another seller really wanted to sell his coastal California practice. He was sick of the small town and wanted to get back to the Northwest where his family lived. He listed the practice, entertained buyers, and even had a signed letter of intent with the one buyer. Then, the seller talked with his wife. The couple weren't just on different pages, they were on different planets. She loved the town and her status there. She threatened divorce if the doctor sold his practice. The sale never happened.

Here are some simple questions to ask to avoid this mistake:

- Have you talked with your financial advisor or CPA about whether or not you can afford to retire?
- How does your spouse feel about selling the practice?

Mistake #2 - Selling the Cow and Trying to Keep the Milk

Many sellers will try to do a delayed sale in which the seller keeps her position in the practice for several months or even years after selling the practice to another owner. I'm generally nervous about delayed sales. I've seen too many deals fall apart and go poorly with much heartache on the buyer's end.

An owner of a practice in Utah thought she was ready to sell. She was the third-generation owner of a practice where she was the main source of production, and her father (the previous owner) was the associate now working two days a week. The practice grossed $1.3 Million in annual collections, and they were asking top dollar for the practice. Our client looked at the numbers with our help, and concluded the price, while steep, was doable. The problem came when negotiations started. The seller wanted an *eight-year guarantee* she would remain employed by the practice with a minimum guaranteed salary, and wanted her father to be contractually guaranteed his current job as associate. The deal never materialized. Clearly, the owner and her family wanted to cash out of the practice, while still being guaranteed an income stream from the business, whether or not the new owner could afford it.

Another orthodontist thought she was ready to sell. Her practice grossed just under $1 Million in collections per year, with good profitability. This seller asked to be kept on the practice, under contract, for 10 years at a per diem of $1,750 a day for a minimum 120 days per year. Clearly the owner wasn't ready to retire or let go. I never could figure out how the seller thought others would think this was a good idea.

Interestingly, both doctors in the examples above were "financially set" and could afford to sell and walk away. Emotionally, however, neither were ready to let go. Both made unreasonable demands that sank the deal. It's not unreasonable for the seller to stick around for a little while after a sale. In most cases, it's preferable to help smooth the transition. The problem comes when "a little while" goes longer than a few months post-transition.

Make sure the seller has something to retire "to" and not just retire "from."

Here are some simple questions to ask to avoid this mistake:

- What are your plans after the sale? Do you want to continue to practice dentistry, and if yes, in what capacity?

- Why do you want to retire?

Mistake #3 - Getting Married Without Dating

I recommend against buying into a partnership or group practice without the opportunity to work alongside your future partner(s). Partnerships are like a second marriage. Even if you will eventually buy out the other doctor, so much rides on working well together. So why would a seller bring someone into the practice without working with them first?

Some sellers believe they need a second set of hands to grow the practice and look around for an associate. They then think they will sell half (or some other percentage) of the practice to a younger dentist, who will then become the partner and eventually buy them all the way out of the business. Then they start looking for a "good" associate. Several interview, a few come visit and maybe even a couple work in the practice. However, finding a good associate turns out to be tougher than they imagined. Some sellers mentally give up and just want to move on. After seeing, interviewing and working with so many associates they get lazy, engage a broker and try and sell half the business to a doctor they've never met or worked with.

This is like an arranged marriage – getting married without ever having dated. The results are predictable in a dental office.

One doctor, after having two associates come and go, decided he needed to sell part of his practice that collected $1.5 Million. He wasn't ready to retire, and was proud of the business he'd built. He thought he would be a great mentor to a new dentist. Having had two "bad" associate experiences ("*bad*" in this case being defined as, "*They didn't want to work the rest of their career at 35% of production and make me rich.*") he wasn't willing to try and work with another associate on an arrangement that would allow them to buy in later. He wanted someone to buy in *now.* He met our client. They hit it off. They compared skills, and everything looked good. They discussed treatment philosophy, and couldn't have been happier with the discussions. They talked about the future plans for the business, and thought they must have been identical twins separated at birth. So, they did the deal. Within 12 months, both doctors realized they weren't a "good fit." The partnership ended in a bitter dispute. Patients left the practice. Employees left to find a more stable environment. The legal bills were huge.

The moral of the story? Never enter a long-term partnership without an acceptable associate term, which allow both parties the chance to work together, judge each other's clinical and managerial abilities, as well as personality fit. There are many ways to work with attorneys to make sure both parties have skin in the game, as well as a way out if an associate-to-own deal doesn't work.

Here are some simple questions to ask to avoid this mistake:

- Have you had associates or partners in the past? Why haven't they stayed?
- Assuming we can align incentives, would you be willing to delay the partnership sale slightly to ensure our works styles and skills are a good fit?

Mistake #4 – Not Putting Things in Writing

Some doctors are very, shall we say…thrifty? They don't want to pay attorneys or accountants, if possible. They assume two reasonable people can come to an agreement, shake hands, and everyone will be fine. This approach ignores human nature, imperfect memories, unsaid assumptions and a host of other potential issues can, and frequently do, come up in transitions.

A doctor was working with a potential associate to whom he intended to eventually sell the practice. The associate engaged me, and I recommended valuing the practice up front and working with legal counsel to draft an employment agreement so everyone's interests were protected. The seller worked hard to convince the buyer, our client, that "his word was his bond" and they didn't need to "waste" money on paying other people as long as they were both upfront, honest and open in their communications. Against my advice, the buyer began working as an associate without any formal agreement on buy out timing or price. A year later, when the buyer was ready to purchase, the seller starting having a few "changes of heart." Conversations the buyer was sure they'd had, were remembered differently by both parties. The seller suddenly wanted more money than they had originally agreed to. The buyer ultimately walked away, and bought another practice. Both the seller and buyer lost a year of their time, money and effort with nothing to show. All to save a few bucks on formalizing an agreement.

Here are some simple questions to ask to avoid this mistake are:

- Who have you engaged to help with this transition? How are they paid?
- How can we be sure to protect ourselves and our interests, and ensure a smooth transition for patients and staff?
- Will you have any issues if I engage my own accountant and lawyer to advise me?

Mistake #5 – Trying to Do It All Yourself

This mistake is a cousin to mistake #4 and a continuation of the do-it-yourself mentality that can carry into business ownership. Every dentist I've met is intelligent. I'm sure you're one of them. You've worked incredibly hard to get where you are, and most of the way when you found an obstacle you learned what you needed to learn and found a way through it.

When it comes time to buy a practice the same attitude that got you into dental school and past those hairy tests kicks in. The dentists about to make this mistake looks around at the steps needed to buy a practice and says, "I can figure this out." And here's the trickiest part of this mistake: You *can* figure it all out.

Unfortunately, it will take you far longer to figure it all out yourself, and if you make any mistakes along the way the impact is usually disastrous. Trying to do it all yourself ignores the principle of treating your time as an asset.

You will be far better off spending your time performing dentistry, improving your clinical skills, or becoming a better manager than you would if you tried to become a practice transition expert, accountant, lawyer, valuation specialist, broker and leasing agent for your own deal.

Personally, as a dental advisor I have learned from experience I need to attach real value to my time. I should spend my time on the activities that either make me money or bring non-monetary fulfillment like time with my family, exercise, mountain biking, and Star Wars movies. And I need to delegate the rest.

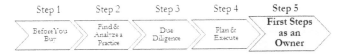

Step 1   Step 2   Step 3   Step 4   Step 5

Before You Buy | Find & Analyze a Practice | Due Diligence | Plan & Execute | First Steps as an Owner

• Hire Good Financial Help
• Change Nothing
• Protect Yourself
• Stick to One Practice

STEP 5:
FIRST STEPS AS AN OWNER

Obviously, this is not a book about practice management, and I'll cover very little about what it takes to be a successful practice owner. However, I have seen common themes and behaviors of those dentists who make a great transition to ownership. Here are a few tips on some of the best first steps you can take as an owner.

Hire Good Financial Help

As a dentist, more than almost any other profession in the country, you understand the value of a quality referral. You know that sometimes the most effective way to help a patient is to get that person to a specialist. The specialist wins and is able to do what they're trained to do, the patient wins as the best person to do the work helps them, and you win as you're able to free up your time to see other patients with problems you can solve.

I recommend following the same principle with your

finances. As the CEO of your dental business, you should outsource the day-to-day management of your finances to a specialist. Don't just hire any accountant. Make sure you hire an accountant that specializes in dental practices.

There are three key reasons for this advice. First, as discussed above, it frees up your time and mental energy and allows you to focus on the thing you do best— dentistry. Don't forget that time you or your staff spend on bookkeeping, payroll, taxes, and other financial projects is time not spent serving and creating a first-class experience for patients.

Second, good accounting keeps you in compliance with the IRS and other governing authorities. A dental accounting specialist ensures you are following the law. Good accounting helps you sleep at night knowing you'll never pay a fine, never go to jail for breaking the rules or underpaying taxes, and (should it occur) could have an auditor in and out of your business in record time.

Third, the monitoring and safeguards in place will protect you and your hard-earned investment from embezzlement. Embezzlement is a real problem in dental offices. 40% of dental offices are victims of embezzlement at some point.

I worked with a client named Mike who dealt with this issue. Statistics show you know someone like Mike.

Mike had over $250,000 stolen from his dental practice over the period of several years by his office manager and most trusted employee, Deb.

Mike contacted me after Deb was charged with embezzlement from a previous job and Mike started to dig into his own numbers. While looking at his past tax returns it was easy to spot where Deb had hidden the money and how she had committed the fraud. Over four years Deb had charged over $250,000 to her own credit card and paid it off using Mike's operating account.

Deb, who was also the "front desk accountant" (kept Quickbooks for Mike), conveniently coded all these payments to "Lab Expense." During these four years, Mike's "Lab Expense" totaled more than 25% of collections. I noticed the problem almost immediately because I knew 5% of collections is a more typical lab expense number. Deb could steal the money and cover her tracks in the books. Mike's local CPA, who handled the finances before I came on the scene, didn't specialize in dentistry and was oblivious to what lab expenses should be and therefore didn't ask any questions.

Embezzlement doesn't happen because dentists are dumb. Mike, like so many others, was actually pretty smart.

Mike was an excellent dentist clinically, personable and well-liked by his patients. He was even smart enough to figure out QuickBooks himself and do his own accounting for a while before delegating this job to Deb.

Mike lost $250,000 because he had a bad accounting system. A good dental accountant will set up a good accounting system.

Dental Accountants Provide Financial Imaging

A good dental accountant can provide financial imaging for your practice that a local CPA or bookkeeper could never provide. You understand the importance of imaging. You know the decisions you make for a patient depend heavily on the quality of image you have. You can see what's coming for the patient, predict the future and create a treatment plan that helps the patient. The same is true for accounting. Good accounting provides the financial imaging to make good quality financial decisions.

Do you know the optimum percentage to pay for staff and benefits? How do you know if you're paying too much for dental supplies? A dental accountant can and should quickly identify what is happening well (and not so well) in your practice.

A good dental accountant takes the non-essential financial tasks off your plate, keeps you in legal compliance with the IRS and others, protects you from thieves, and more. The real power of accounting lies in the ability to make good business decisions.

The First 90 Days – Change Nothing

Maybe it's because the press write news stories about new CEOs or Presidents and the "first 90 days" that makes new dentists think they have to make some dramatic change when they first buy their practice. After analyzing and doing due diligence on the practice you're buying, you'll likely see things you want to change in the practice right away.

Don't do it.

I'm serious. Don't change a thing for at least 90 days. If you're buying a practice, you ostensibly bought it because it has some value and some redeeming qualities. The very worst thing you can do as a new owner of an existing dental practice is to change things. The staff and patients are already coping with a change in the boss. Even if they're excited to have you on board, you're still largely an unknown, with all the disruption, stress, and anxiety that brings.

Changing anything to do with the staff is a mistake in the first few months. For them, you are now the person with a big neon flashing sign over your head that says, "Watch out! I control your addiction to food, clothing and shelter and could fire you." I generally try to avoid comparing dental teams to families, but in this case the comparison is useful. Imagine you have a family with one child. That's three relationships. Now add a new baby. Now you have six relationships, most of which are now changed and different. The oldest child now has competition for attention. Mom and Dad now have three people to think about, instead of two. New people cause a lot of disruption.

Now think of the size of a dental team. And don't limit the numbers to just the staff. Think about all the vendors and suppliers. Referral doctor relationships will change. Patients' relationships will need to be rebuilt.

After all this, to add new processes, priorities, goals and procedures is ludicrous. Don't do it.

Learn, ask questions, fit in. Find out why they do things the way they do. Take notes, build relationships, and listen. The time to change will come.

Over the first 90 days if you make your focus on learning and fitting in, and not "fixing this broken practice so it can achieve its full potential (and make me rich)" a remarkable thing will happen. You'll understand better *why* they've been doing what they're doing and you'll have much better relationships to make the changes you still feel you need to change after your first few months.

Protect Yourself with Insurance

Most new dentists are relatively unfamiliar with the various types of insurance policies needed as a practice owner. Insurance exists to protect you from something catastrophic that could ruin you financially. Yes, insurance will cost money. If you're a newer dentist you may be reluctant to spend money on insurance. That reluctance is a mistake. While it is possible to overpay for insurance, paying for insurance will rarely, if ever, make a dent in your long-term financial goals. But not having insurance and needing it can derail your entire financial future.

There are dozens of different insurance policies you could get as a business owner. Your goal is to insure against events that you cannot afford to have happen. You should be aware of a few of the most common and useful types of insurance for practice owners. Be sure you work with a qualified and trusted resource to help you evaluate the insurance you'll need in your new practice. I recommend you protect yourself and your investment in a new practice with the insurance policies listed below.

Professional Liability Insurance (Malpractice)

Malpractice coverage is for individuals, corporations, or employees and covers damages for a variety of professional liability incidents. A policy can also cover hygienists and assistants employed in your office. You can buy a "claims policy" at a discount rate when you're first getting started, and may consider purchasing an "occurrence" policy. Both protect against you as a medical professional and have slightly different rules about when coverage kicks in. A discounted claims policy will cost about a few hundred a year for a recent graduate, but rates will increase after five years and will generally be higher in metro areas.

Workers Compensation Insurance

Workers compensation insurance is generally mandatory for all offices and the requirements will vary from state to state. Usually this will be set up automatically with the help of your payroll company as you get set up, but be sure to ask so that you are compliant with your state's regulations. These rates are set by your state.

Business Contents Insurance

Business contents insurance covers general liability, office furnishings, equipment, building improvements to leased space and build-outs. Can include business income accounts receivable and wind/hail coverage. Rates are determined by location and amount of property protected by the policy.

General Liability Insurance

General liability insurance covers practices to protect them against claims for bodily injury and property damage that happen at your office, from normal business operations and products of the dental practice. Rates are determined by location and risk factors determined by the insurance company.

Umbrella or Excess Liability

Umbrella insurance provides extra coverage in the event of claim loss in excess of underlying policy limits. For example, you are sued for $2 Million, but your malpractice coverage only covers claims up to $1 Million. Umbrella can cover general liability, employer's liability, and auto insurance liability and other types of policies.

Disability Insurance

Disability insurance exists to protect you in case you have a physical or medical problem that prevents you from practicing dentistry. You should consider three different types of disability coverage.

The first type is Income Replacement disability insurance. This will be the type of disability coverage with the longest term and will protect you until you retire, or can afford to self-insure. Income replacement disability coverage typically covers up to 60% of your income, and can be written to protect you until you reach retirement age. The amount you actually need will depend greatly on how much you spend each month, if your spouse works, and what you want to do if you can't practice dentistry.

The second type of disability insurance you should consider is business loan protection coverage. This type of insurance will cover your practice loan payments if you become disabled before you pay off the loan. The policy will be tied directly to a specific loan, and would be paid directly to the bank in the case of disability. Because the coverage is for the term of the loan, it can be cheaper to protect your loan obligations this way compared to using your income replacement coverage.

The third type of disability coverage to consider is business overhead expense coverage. This coverage reimburses you for business expenses like utilities, employees, rent and other expenses you would want to cover for a short-term disability situation, where you are planning to return to dentistry.

Every situation is unique and every person's needs are different, so it is hard to give blanket advice to everyone reading this as to which disability insurance policy or policies they should have. I recommend knowing the options and considering each of the three types at a minimum.

Life Insurance

Life insurance is not really for you. Life insurance protects the people who depend on your pay as a dentist. If you die prematurely, life insurance provides your family with the income stream they would have received if you were around.

Life insurance needs to be part of your financial plan. But, it should not be the plan itself. The two types of life insurance you'll need to decide between are term and whole life insurance. If you're just buying your practice, especially if you're early in your career, I recommend you buy term and not whole life insurance.

I can hear the whole life insurance zealots now, "Whole life offers great returns!" and "It's much safer than the stock market!" I've heard it all before. Every time I sit and analyze a client's whole life policy they've been paying on for several years, what they were *told* they would have in their account is never even close to what they *actually* have.

The differences in a nutshell are basic. Term insurance is a monthly bill you pay, hoping you never see any benefit. (Because you're not dead! That's good!) Whole life insurance is also a monthly bill, but instead of never seeing your money again if you don't die, when you're *much* older, the policy has a cash value you can then borrow from, withdraw, pass on to heirs, etc.

The first reason you should lean towards term insurance is cost. I ran a quote on myself for a $2.5-million-dollar term life policy. (For the record, I'm in my mid 30's, and a non-smoker.) The cost was $1,760/year. I then ran a quote for a whole life policy worth $250,000 (10% of the amount my wife would get if I die, compared to the term policy.) The cost was $3,440/year. This is double the cost for 10% of the benefit with whole life. Term insurance is always <u>much</u> cheaper. The brutal fact is that in order to be adequately covered, you'll probably need a large amount of coverage. If you feel better with a whole life policy, the cost to get to that big number becomes so prohibitive, most choose inadequate coverage and their dependents suffers as a result.

The second reason to choose term insurance is that term is straightforward and easy to understand. One thing that drives financial advisors like me up the wall is when we see the assumptions in the presentation given to dentists about choosing a whole life policy. So often the assumptions are not realistic. It would be like an orthodontist walking in and telling a patient they can permanently straighten their teeth in two months for $250. As a new dentist, you don't know the finer points of life insurance and investment assumptions. Why would you? Just like I don't know one dentist's choice to choose a cheap composite on my filling was a poor choice, often times I see people making poor decisions about insurance based on assumptions that are very unrealistic. Term insurance is simple. Pay a small premium, and if you die, your heirs get a big check. That's it. Simpler is better here.

The third reason to choose term insurance is that choosing term doesn't confuse insurance with an investment. Insurance is a transference of risk. You transfer the risk over many people like you, which reduces everyone's risk. When you try to overlay investments on top of that, it gets exponentially more expensive. Keep your insurance in its own lane, and keep investments in their own lane. Besides, as a new practice owner, chances are you're more focused on increasing your earnings and paying down debt.

Investing serious amounts of money probably won't come for at least a few years into your career.

The fourth and final reason to choose term life insurance is that the commissions are cheaper. Commissions on insurance policies can run anywhere from 55% to 100% of the first year's premium. You saw how differently term and whole life policies get priced with my own example. Thus, human nature being what it is, your insurance agent has a strong incentive to sell you the more expensive policy. Not every insurance agent will push you towards an inferior option. In fact, I work closely with several insurance agents I know and trust. However, I've seen the results of enough poorly understood and poorly placed whole life policies that I know bad actors are out there.

While it's true that I rarely recommend whole life for my clients, there can be situations where it makes sense. Typically, whole life insurance has a place in the portfolios of high-earners who have maxed out their other investment opportunities and are looking for an ultra-conservative place to invest.

Many financial advisors and dental accountants love whole life because of the income it provides *their* business. The numbers have not worked for my clients. I recommend term life insurance as the best option for dentists—especially new ones.

Plan to Only Buy One Practice

This will be the most controversial section in the book. The advice here runs contrary to the popular advice today in the dental world. I'm sure you've heard the message: If owning one practice is good, two is better, and three or more is best. "You're a chump and failed dentist if you only own one dental practice," is the clear message. You'll hear the advice to own multiple practices throughout your career from all sides.

The sad truth is that owning multiple practices is tougher than most believe. Owning multiple practices most often leads to more headaches, more stress, more debt, more risk, and less income for the owner.

Advocates for the multi-practice model tend to ignore the fact that dental practice costs are mostly fixed, requiring much more work, energy, and effort for more money when compared to growing one practice. Also, finding a good long-term associate is much more difficult than people assume. Finally, the skillset needed to run a large organization is very different than the one needed to run one practice.

Dental Practice Costs are Mostly Fixed

The average doctor might say her overhead is 65%. That is true, but incomplete. And very misleading. Of the 65% number only 15% is variable costs, and the remaining 50% are fixed costs.

And in any business you don't make any money until you cover your fixed costs!

Let's assume you own a practice collecting $1 Million annually, and you have overhead totaling 65%—15%

variable and 50% fixed. You keep $350k currently and let's assume you want to make $100,000 more next year.

One way to do it would be to increase your collections in your existing practice. Your variable expenses would increase, but the total increase you'll need to see in your practice collections to make another $100,000 is $117,647.

What if, instead, you decide to open a second location. How much more will you need to collect to make that extra $100,000?

Your fixed costs will double with the second location. Now, you'll need to collect an additional $705,882 to make an additional $100,000. Don't forget you're running two practices now instead of one, with all the associated debt, stress, and risk.

(Figure 5.1)

Making an Additional $100,000 Illustration

	Current Practice	Increase Collections	Buy a Second Practice
Collections	$1,000,000	$1,117,647	$1,705,882
Variable Costs (15%)	$150,000	$167,647	$255,882
Fixed Costs (50%)	$500,000	$500,000	$1,000,000
Total Overhead	$650,000	$667,647	$1,255,882
Operating Income	$350,000	$450,000	$450,000

Which option seems easier to you?

"But wait!" you say, "I'll have an associate running the other practice!"

Finding a Good Associate is a Lot Harder Than You Expect

Dentists who think they'll find great associates who want to work hard to make them rich, forget that when they were an associate they were already looking for the exit, planning their own practice purchase.

The good dentists that you'd be willing to hire? They don't want to work for you. They want to own their practice just like you.

So what ends up happening is these practice owners are constantly recruiting the next associate because the last good one just left. You should know. You were that good associate now buying a practice.

Ask yourself this question: What percentage of your graduating dental school class would you be willing to partner with, hire, borrow hundreds of thousands of dollars to employ, and put your reputation on the line for?

I'm willing to bet the percentage in your head isn't large. But for some reason when you start a second practice you think it will magically be run by great associates.

Good luck.

You're Not Very Good at Running Large Businesses

Some dentists make a very dangerous leap of logic. They think to themselves, "Running one practice is easy! Running two or more can't be much harder."

While it's possible you could be the exception, most dentists barely get by on the organizational skills required to run one practice. Managing a large organization requires a very different skill set than being a good dentist in one practice.

All of this doesn't mean owning multiple practice locations won't work for you. You could be the exception.

If your lifelong dream is to build a dental empire and one day sell your conglomerate to a private equity firm and retire a billionaire, I wish you success.

Having more locations guarantees an increase in the amount of money your accountant, lawyer, consultants, equipment and supply reps, and banker make. Perhaps that's one of the reasons the advice to buy a second practice is so prevalent?

If, however, you got into dentistry to build a great life helping others, improving health, making good money all with some balance in life, plan on owning one practice and making it great.

Get Help!

I would love to work directly with you.

Get a FREE phone consultation about your specific situation or find out about working directly with me.

Email Me Directly:
Brian@BrianHanks.com

Or Visit **www.BrianHanks.com**

Made in the USA
Middletown, DE
04 March 2019